IF NOT NOW, WHEN?

THE RETIREMENT GUIDE YOU'VE BEEN WAITING FOR

Ginni Gordon

First edition June 2017
Printed and bound in the United States of America
ISBN: 978-0-692-90152-6

I dedicate this book,
with love and so much appreciation
to the wonderful friends that rose up,
held my hand, cracked the whip
and kept me at task, until we were done.

I couldn't have done it alone…
and I am so grateful I didn't have to.

FOREWORD

I began my own retirement process in 2001 and, at that time, I experienced what I call the "What's Next" phenomenon. One of my past careers was to lead parents through the process of working with their teenagers who were experiencing drug and alcohol problems. It taught me to work with people and counsel them through difficult times. I discovered that these procedures can be used with other challenges and that they actually work well in the area of dealing with retirement. The techniques that helped me to guide others during this season of their life can assist and support retirees on both an experiential and an emotional level.

This book is for people who are entering the retirement phase of their lives and are not quite sure what to do next. Or maybe they are just looking for something new to enrich this time of their life. I have drawn the strategies described in it from my own life experiences, putting into practice the "Letting Go" process and putting these experiences to good use in new adventures.

This book offers a comprehensive, step-by-step process to explore "life after retirement." It is easy to follow and describes how to turn retirement into an adventure filled with enjoyment and satisfaction. The book includes exercises that encourage the reader to "think outside the box," to put the philosophy of this book into action and adapt the skills acquired from their past accomplishments into "What's next." After all, this is *your time*, and like the title says, "If Not Now, When?"

Group seminars are available to assist in putting these concepts into action.
Contact Ginni Gordon at retireifnotnowwhen@yahoo.com

TABLE OF CONTENTS

To be happy, you must:
1) Let go of what's gone.
2) Be grateful for what remains.
3) Look forward to what's to come.
    —Unknown

INTRODUCTION

One day, you will wake up and there
won't be any more time to do the things
you've always wanted. Do it now.
—Paulo Coelho

Back in the day, when I first retired, I experienced a sense of freedom, a sense of not having my life based on making my extracurricular activities fit into a certain time frame. After a month or so, I realized that I had not really thought this process through and was left feeling like I was in a rowboat without any oars. I had little idea what I was "supposed" to do next and what I really wanted from the future. What was missing, for me, was a purpose and a plan for the transition from working to retirement. I even needed to define, for myself, what retirement really meant.

I eventually discovered that it is possible to retire and create a meaningful life. I have learned to creatively use the time that was taken up by my career to explore "what's next?" and "what do I want now?" because, as the title of the book says, "If not now, when?" I found the skills I had accumulated over the years were transferable into other areas of my life, and that gave my existence purpose and meaning.

I interviewed a number of retirees for this book and discovered that many of them had also encountered difficulties navigating this process. For some of them, the interviews we did were, in a way, cathartic. Telling their story helped to put the process in perspective. Some people I talked to related that they had postponed their retirement because they didn't know "what they would do with themselves." I also discovered that being retired is as different, for each person, as the people are themselves. I have included some personal experiences and some interviews with retirees who have chosen different ways to express this time in their lives. And, although all our experiences may differ, having a guide through the process can save a lot of time, angst and frustration.

Initially, retirement can seem like a puzzle with many pieces to be put into the appropriate places. Sometimes the exact position can seem obscure until a few experiences (puzzle parts) fit together and the picture starts to take shape. And, when you put enough of the puzzle/experience together, you then see the space that is left to be worked with. I have met retirees that have moved into amazingly creative places, doing things they had never imagined they would do. This book is designed to guide you through the process of putting together the puzzle pieces of retirement. It will help you ask the questions you might not have even thought about; I sure know I hadn't. One of my favorite questions has become, "If Not Now, When?" Thus the name of this book and a reason to not let opportunities go to waste.

The decision to turn the question, "If not now, when?" into a book was made when I was on a Mediterranean cruise with my friend Diane Askew. We had been chatting about the possibility of someday writing a book. I shared with her how thought-provoking I considered this question and how it had helped me make decisions to get into action in several areas. While we were in a bookstore in a small town in Spain, she discovered a journal with lined pages. Printed on the cover were the words, "If Not Now, When?" When she handed it to me she said, "I think you are supposed to write this book."

When I returned home, I enrolled in a weekend seminar presented by Mary Morrissey called "Dream Builder's Workshop." This wonderful program let me develop and work on my decision to go forward with this project, to actually picture it manifesting into form. I have included some of her inspiring quotes throughout this book and in the reading list at the end.

I heard about and enrolled in an online book-writing class, Writer's Workshop Forum, presented by the pastor of my church, Dr. James Turrell, and his partner, Lee Pound. With the guidance of their wonderful program, I was able to create this book, one paragraph at a time. I have included information about this class, for those of you who think this could be something you would enjoy, in the resource section at the end of this book. I also received valuable assistance from Anne Perrah and John Lunsford, both published authors. Their coaching and advice took me over more than a few rough spots.

The "You" of you is not
the "You" of your credentials.
If, however, you are stuck
in your personal history,
you may become a
"credential collector"
—believing that you are defined
by your business card
and degrees.
Instead, attune yourself to
the inner voice whispering,
"Wake up! It's time to be free
and step into your true identity
as an evolving being."
—Michael Bernard Beckwith

The book is set up in such a way that you will be an active participant. I have included "homework" at the end of each chapter that will encourage you to take on this investigation into your future. You will begin with an examination of your career and what leaving it behind means to you. This will include delving into the feelings that arise and the possible need to grieve the sense of loss that is there for many of us at this time. You will also investigate the expertise you have amassed and how those skills can be used elsewhere.

You will examine the phenomenon of being a beginner in life—again; what it's going to take to move forward and all the wonderful skills that will accompany this process. You will also be watching out for any "self-talk" that might try to sabotage you at this point: statements like "I'm too old" or "That is just going to take too long" or "I don't want to start over again; it's too much work." These all floated through my mind at one time.

You may consider continuing to work part-time, possibly doing something interesting you wouldn't have considered before. And, you will look at taking your talents into the area of service work, of "paying it forward." I recently read that there is a plethora of wonderfully talented seniors who are and can be contributing to others. Doing this kind of work has been, to me, meaningful beyond words. I am presently acting, singing and dancing in a musical filled with Broadway songs. I would have never thought of doing this if I hadn't had the time to work on these skills. And most of the performances we do are for senior organizations and veterans; they make great audiences.

You will also be encouraged to start a bucket list (if you haven't already done so). I hadn't, and I find that having this open-ended list provides a place for me to write whatever pops into my mind. You will also develop skills that will assist you in trying new things and a way to recognize how the talents you have amassed in past accomplishments make doing new things much easier.

Please have a notebook/journal handy for a few of the "homework assignments"; this will give you a chance to be a "hands on" participant in this process of life change. You are encouraged to do the exercises; you will be surprised at what is still left to learn about you. Know for a fact that the future most likely holds many experiences that will bring joy and meaning to you. The choice of how you spend this time is completely in your hands.

Note: When you find an author's name in **bold**, *this is your indication that there is a book by this author listed in the Recommended Reading List (p. 113).*

CHAPTER 1
BACK IN THE DAY...

When one door closes, another opens.
But we often look so long and so regretfully
upon the closed door that we do not see
the one that has opened for us.
—Alexander Graham Bell

WHO AM I, AND WHAT DO I DO NOW, HAVE NOW, GET TO BE NOW?

So, you have retired. Or maybe you are just entering the conversation about starting this part of your life. The first part of your time off may be spent having the adventures you promised yourself, like those golf games on weekdays and the lengthy vacations you always wanted to take. I have also had people tell me they spent some of this time "putting their house in order": doing the repairs that have been waiting patiently to be attended to. After "living the life you richly deserve," much to your surprise, boredom can set in. The joy, excitement, and freedom you expected to feel disappear, and you can find you have lost your "purpose" for getting up in the morning. I know; it happened that way for me... all except the weekly golf games.

Many retired people, or those who plan on retirement in the near future, discover that their careers, education, and life roles are how they have chosen to judge their self-worth. They often find themselves experiencing the "who am I?" and "what do I do now?" stage of their life. So, ask yourself these questions:

WHO AM I? AND WHAT DO I WANT TO DO WITH THE REST OF MY LIFE?

With time on your hands, you may find yourself facing the fear of the unknown. You may spend time hiding out in the past ("How wonderful my life was when I became president of my company!"), feeling your life has lost its meaning, and asking yourself, "Is that all there is . . . for me?"

This book is designed to help you navigate through this time. We will look at where you are coming from (your career/education/job titles) and introduce a process that lets you examine what is truly there for you in your future. This is a period in which you can decide to change your identity, discover who you thought you were, and entertain the possibility of developing a whole new you.

Life as we knew it is passing away,
and something new is emerging
to take its place.
—Marianne Williamson

I have included interviews with people who have retired and made a variety of different choices. There is no "right" choice; you will find that there are many different ways to go. I have also discovered there is no such thing as a "retiree"; we are all as different as our lives and our stories. This gives you the immense freedom to create your life to be what you want it to be.

When I made up my mind to retire from my job as a dental hygienist, I went into the doctors' office (my dentist bosses were also my brothers) and told them of my plans. As we crowded into their small office space, the tension inside me grew. I wondered how they were going to receive my news. The office was filled with overstuffed chairs and a large oak desk; dusty textbooks lined the walls. The small glow from the X-ray viewer did its best to add some light to the room. My brother Jim and I took the seats facing the desk, while my brother Larry sat across from us.

I cleared my throat and told them about my plans to retire. I assured them that this wasn't going to be one of those "two weeks' notice" endings. After all, we had been in practice together for 25 years. As a matter of fact, the retirement process took me over nine months. One of my biggest obstacles to retiring was dealing with patients who didn't want me to leave. My most devoted patients seemed to think I had magical powers that helped them keep their mouths healthy.

I discovered that people get just as attached to their hygienist as they do to their hairstylist. They enjoyed the connection with a hygienist who remembered them and what was going on in their lives, and I loved hearing what was new for them. There were feelings of loyalty on both sides. I used a lot of humor to keep my patients comfortable. While sitting in my chair to have his teeth cleaned, one man told me that I was going to be "mad at him" because he hadn't been flossing. I told him that I already had four kids and wasn't going to adopt him, so the responsibility for his oral health was his. I took advantage of the remaining few visits with my apprehensive patients to introduce them to one of the other hygienists and reassured them that they would be well taken care of.

When I had finished the retirement process, my brothers sold the practice, and a new dentist took over the office. He enjoyed having me on hand as a fill-in—and for me, having the ability to be at the office softened the shock of being retired. Yes, it was quite a shock. This office, and the room in which I took care of my patients, had always seemed like my second home. It now belonged to another hygienist.

I had expected life to go on as it had been; I am a busy person who likes to be involved in activities. But once my retirement was complete, I found myself jumping out of bed, brushing my teeth (and flossing, of course), getting dressed, going downstairs to have breakfast and realizing that I had gotten "all dressed up with no place to go." I quickly realized I needed to look at where my life was going next.

What I judged as missing, for me, was a purpose and a plan for the transition from working to retirement. While some may consider "work" a four-letter word, many of us see our careers as challenging, fulfilling, and enriching.

First, I needed to decide what, for me, retirement really meant. I eventually did discover—over a period of time and with much "research and development"—that it is possible to retire and still have a meaningful life. I have learned to creatively use the time that was taken up by my career to explore "what's next" and "what do I want my life to be like now?" I have also discovered that there is more room available in my schedule to try on different experiences. You may just discover that your life becomes something you could not have imagined even in your wildest dreams. Mine did.

AM I SOLELY DEFINED BY MY CAREER, LIFE ROLES, DEGREES, BY WHOM THE WORLD SEES ME TO BE?

You can't start the next
chapter of your life
if you keep rereading
the last one.
—Unknown

Many people who are retiring from their careers discover that they are not prepared for the emotional consequences that follow this dramatic change. Quite often, they have spent a lot of time and education developing their occupation, and retirement can feel like a type of death. It's true: giving up the part of yourself that made you feel valuable can create an empty void. The fear that arises at this point can put you in a place where you don't want to move forward, where you feel frozen in time.

David Whyte, author of *Crossing the Unknown Sea*, describes it this way: "Sometimes we have built walls around ourselves, and they served to shelter us at certain periods of our life only to imprison us when we have remained within their confines too long. Our work emboldens us for a while, and then, if we do not invigorate and reimagine our participation, it begins to enclose us and slowly starve our spirit. Good work done in the same way for too long eats away at your sense of being right with the world."

If you hold the belief that "I Have Done It All" and "My Best Days Are Behind Me," it can leave you with no place to go. If you hold the belief that you have already accomplished all of your life goals, you can truly be in a place with nowhere to turn. If you don't want to start over as a "beginner" in life, your focus will often center on "what I used to do" and "who I used to be" and not on "what new experiences I can now have and what new things I can start incorporating into my life." With this frame of mind, you will have a lot of "back in the day" conversations, and your discussions will usually center on your past accomplishments.

I have discovered that it's hard to move forward if you feel you have already accomplished all of your objectives in life. I discovered, during my research, a number of people who felt just this way when they considered retirement.

So, pause here for a moment and ask yourself this question:

"Do I believe that I have already done in life all I set out to do?"

(Make a few notes about your initial reaction/evaluation of where you see yourself in regard to this question right now.)

HAVE I DONE IT ALL?

_____

_____

_____

_____

_____

_____

_____

_____

I grew up in a family that valued "left brain" pursuits. Both my brothers graduated from University of Southern California School of Dentistry, and I graduated as a dental hygienist from the University of California, Los Angeles (USC's rival). I spent much of my life seeking out education in areas I found interesting. Besides being a hygienist, I have a teaching credential in health sciences at the college/university level. I have taught at USC, UCLA, and Cerritos and Saddleback community colleges. I also ran parent groups for families whose children were experiencing drug and alcohol problems and eating disorders. I am currently a licensed practitioner at the Center for Spiritual Living Newport-Mesa.

For a while after I retired, my "right brain" demanded its turn, and I found myself drawn to more creative pursuits. I began by performing in dance groups and taking up photography. I had taken tap dancing for many years, as much for the exercise as for the fun. This skill led me to be a little courageous and to start performing in shows. As scared as I was at first, my love of dancing propelled me forward. Later I studied Polynesian dance, and that took me even further toward overcoming my fear of being on stage.

In May 2012, a good friend saw an ad in *The Orange County Register* for participants over 60 to enter the Ms. Senior Orange County Pageant. She convinced me we should try out and do it together. You need to understand that I am *not* a pageant woman; I had never done anything like this in my life. We had a meeting with the pageant director, and she accepted us as contestants. The pageant was to take place exactly two weeks later.

I scrambled around, found a long dress in the closet (for the modeling section), picked out a dance I had done a number of times as a solo ("Keep Your Eyes on the Hands," a fun Hawaiian hula) and came up with a "Philosophy of Life" that had to be presented in under 35 seconds. Luckily, senior women weren't required to compete in a bikini. Then, a few days before the pageant, my friend dropped out of the competition.

The day before the pageant dawned, and I showed up along with the other 19 women in the contest. We rehearsed our talks and the numbers we had chosen to perform. The next day the show went off without a hitch; I didn't have time to get nervous (remember, no bikini competition—and my expectations were low). To my surprise, I won. I am, and always will be, Ms. Senior Orange County 2012. The pictures following my crowning are hilarious; many of them show me with my mouth hanging open in surprise.

Through this experience, I met wonderful women who inspire me to keep "taking the next step." A group of us perform variety shows for many local senior centers and veterans organizations. We have traveled to Las Vegas and Laughlin, Nevada, and to New Orleans to perform during Mardi Gras 2016. Our latest projects have been two musicals. The first one is based on the first 100 years on Broadway and the latest one focuses on the music of Irving Berlin.

IS THIS ALL THERE IS TO LIFE?

You are now at a crossroads.
Forget your past. Who are you now?
Don't think about who you have been.
—Tony Robbins

Right about now you, the retiree, may be wondering, "Is that all there is?" and "If not, what am I going to do now?" You may find yourself thinking, "I knew who I was when I was actively pursuing my career, but who am I now?" It is possible for this time to provide an exciting experience, a chance to take a stab at a whole new way of being. But it can also be a time where people find themselves perplexed, feeling as if their motivation for living has gone.

It is also not unusual to see people at this stage of retirement develop coping mechanisms to prevent their emotions from coming to the surface. One of my first encounters with this retirement phenomenon centered on my Uncle Art. He had a wonderful career as a long-distance truck driver. One of his favorite hauls involved taking missiles from California to Cape Canaveral, a complicated and responsible task. He liked to tell us stories of his trips and the people he met along the way.

He and my Aunt Dinny (short for Virginia) had been married many years and had a wonderful little house in Los Angeles where we attended many fun parties. His personality made him a very popular uncle with all his nieces and nephews. He looked and sounded a lot like Wallace Beery, the old-time movie star. When Uncle Art retired, his attitude toward life changed. He went from being outgoing and merry to sitting in front of the television, focused on whatever was showing.

Aunt Dinny had imagined a different retirement, one in which they would be out and about, going places, and visiting friends. Their daughter, a flight attendant (then called a "stewardess") with TWA, provided many opportunities to travel on her passes. Uncle Art felt he had worked hard, had traveled as many miles and seen as much of the world as he cared to, and was ready to take it easy.

I remember thinking how unfulfilling life seemed for Aunt Dinny and yet, she agreed with Uncle Art that he had, indeed, earned his downtime. After a while, Aunt Dinny found herself visiting with her sisters, and she still had family parties at their house. I saw that you can make life work if that is your intention . . . and I also remember thinking that I wouldn't want to be stuck at home in front of a television for the rest of my life.

Research for this book has led me to several more people with Uncle Art's philosophy. They feel that they have worked hard all their lives, that they have the right to choose how to spend their retirement time, what to eat (ice cream for breakfast, etc.), and whom to hang out with. One man told me, "I am done working; if I need to get something fixed, I call someone on Craigslist." While I agree with a person's right to feel this way, I knew it wasn't how I wanted to spend my remaining years. What's more, in articles I have read, it is estimated that men who retire to a sedentary style of living have an average life expectancy of three years.

I now see retirement as an opportunity to explore all the wonderful things life has to offer—and I know that getting there is truly a process.

For what it's worth . . . it's never too late
to be whoever you want to be.
There's no time limit. Start whenever you want.
You can change or stay the same.
There are no rules to this thing.
We can make the best or the worst of it.
I hope you make the best of it.
I hope you see things that startle you.
I hope you feel things you never felt before.
I hope you meet people who have
a different point of view.
I hope you live a life you're proud of,
and if you're not,
I hope you have the courage
to start all over again.
—Eric Roth,
"The Curious Case of Benjamin Button" Screenplay

Let's look again at the purpose of this book. We are going to take an adventure into the unknown: into Your Future. This is a process that will let you develop a whole new way of thinking/being, while holding onto the wisdom you have collected in the past. You will have the opportunity to discover that much of your life is still left to enjoy: an adventure that's rewarding and fulfilling. **Know that this is a choice.**

As I said, what you want to do with the rest of your life is your choice and your right to decide. If you choose to take this adventure (and maybe just explore other possibilities), you might discover something new about yourself and the possibilities for your future.

BOB ESTRADA'S STORY

When selecting people to interview for this book, I knew right away that I wanted to talk with Bob. I have known Bob and his wife for a number of years. We go to the same church, and I have attended many events at their lovely house. Bob and I decided to meet for our interview at a restaurant. Well, actually at two restaurants. We had so much fun talking, it took a couple of sessions to get all the information I wanted.

Both of us like good food, so we did one meeting at a wonderful Japanese restaurant and the second get-together at an Italian restaurant. Because Bob and I are retired, we had all the time we needed to enjoy the experience of sharing this period of our lives. Choosing Bob appealed to me because he had been retired for a short period of time (less than a year) and because I was so impressed with his transition from a successful career to retirement. His story is interesting and shows his creativity both in his career and his retirement.

For 45 years, Bob centered his employment on one of his greatest loves, automobiles. His jobs were in sales of auto parts and engine lubricants, managing customers, and taking their orders. He was 67 when he retired and it was, as he put it, "my choice." His last job was with a man he respected and enjoyed working for. He had pursued that job for two years and the atmosphere, although it did demand a high level of production, was more in keeping with the kind of man and employee he truly was.

This was not like the job he had before, where he worked with a company whose boss had told him, "We have to keep the pressure up on you guys in order to keep this company profitable." He was part of the staff that transferred after a company acquisition. He always felt that his boss made his job as "miserable as possible," hoping he would quit. Instead, what he did was develop a personal philosophy that he would be the best he could be in any situation. During his employment with this company, he was named Top Salesman of the Year twice.

Bob and his wife, Diane, had taken a dream vacation to Monaco for their 30th wedding anniversary, where they could watch the Grand Prix. They traveled the area in a beautiful clipper ship; it was truly the vacation of a lifetime. He and Diane took some of this time to discuss their future. Diane had recovered from breast cancer, and they both were committed to having a wonderful "rest of their life." Bob made a pledge that, when they returned home, they would live the life of their dreams. They decided that this vacation, rather than being the high point of their lives, was to be a portal to living the rest of their lives at a higher level.

Shortly after they returned, Bob contracted influenza that kept him in bed for three weeks. During this time he still tried to maintain contact with his customers, until his doctor said, "No. Bed rest only, no phones, computers, etc." His boss agreed with the doctor and told him, "Talk to me when you are well." During this down time, he came to the conclusion that the life he wanted for himself and his wife could no longer be based on being a high producer. So, even though he loved his job and his boss, he decided to retire.

He shared with me that, for a period of time after his retirement, he did have what I call the "Limbo Experience." I have heard this reported by a number of people who were recently retired, and I certainly experienced it myself. Although it can present in many different ways, retirement is, for many people, an adjustment into the unknown.

In keeping with their dedication to have the rest of their life be the best part of their life, Bob decided to take a series of classes at our church that would enable him to become a Center of Spiritual Living Licensed Practitioner. This program takes about three years and offers students a chance to grow and deepen in their spirituality and their counseling skills.

Bob and Diane also continued a practice of spending time together in the morning, planning their day in a positive way, praying and acknowledging the things they were grateful for.

Bob shared with me his belief that "Life is constantly conspiring in our favor; our job is to look for evidence of that." Put that together with Abraham Lincoln's belief that "People are generally as happy as they decide to be," and you can see why Bob is a great role model for retirement.

HOMEWORK ASSIGNMENT FOR CHAPTER 1

1. Your first assignment is to make a list of all your careers/jobs, your titles, your roles in life, your volunteer jobs, etc. Place them in single file along the left side of the space below.

When making this list, use your imagination and be creative. For example, you can include things you did in the past that you see yourself possibly doing again in the future.

MY CAREERS / JOBS / LIFE ROLES / TITLES / DEGREES

_____

_____

_____

_____

_____

_____

_____

2. As you read over your list, ask yourself these questions:

▶ "What have I enjoyed most about this career/job I had?"

▶ "What did I like/enjoy least about this career/job I am leaving behind?"

▶ "What aspects of my career/job will I miss the most? What parts of it would I most like to continue doing?"

This exercise will start your imagination working on "What's Next?"

3. Write your realizations on the lines below:

WHAT I LIKED/ENJOYED OR DIDN'T LIKE/ENJOY ABOUT MY CAREERS/JOBS. WHICH ASPECTS WOULD I MISS/ LIKE TO CONTINUE DOING?

_____

_____

_____

_____

_____

_____

ADDITIONAL NOTES

_____

_____

_____

_____

_____

_____

_____

_____

_____

_____

_____

_____

_____

_____

_____

_____

_____

CHAPTER 2
CLEANING OUT THE CUPBOARDS

You are not defined by your past.
You are prepared by your past.
—Joel Osteen

TAKE A LOOK AT YOUR LIST OF CAREERS

So let's get to work!

Open to the homework assignment for Chapter 1 and take a look at the list of your achievements. We're going to examine these careers, titles, and roles you made note of and use them in this next exercise.

With a pencil, cross out any careers, life roles, titles, and degrees that no longer define who you are in the present moment. Recognize that, in reality, you are not going to be completely saying goodbye to any of your accomplishments. What you have achieved will always be a part of you! You will discover this as we continue this process.

Even though this may seem like serious stuff, treat this exercise like a game. There is no wrong way to play it, and you have an eraser on your pencil if you change your mind.

Deciding to start this goodbye/cleaning-out process is a huge hurdle for some. To illustrate how this procedure functions, I use the analogy of cleaning out the cupboards in my kitchen.

As I start on my cupboards, I decide that it doesn't hurt to be aggressive with this "cleaning-out" task. Organizing my cupboards so they'll be shipshape is my primary goal. And because that is true, it's a wonderful feeling to have completed the task. I have learned that the best method is to take everything out of the cupboard, even those items I am sure I want to save. What I have also discovered is that, in order to get the best result, I need to wash the shelves (there's almost always a mystery substance stuck there).

It's not what you look at
that matters,
it's what you see.
—Henry David Thoreau

Then comes the process of throwing out or recycling what I no longer need to keep. This can take some thought. Once in a while, I will want to hold onto an item I have an attachment to: a bowl that a friend gave me, a spice that I enjoy using in a certain dish. At moments like this, I may need to be a bit ruthless. Keeping my goal in mind, that of having a clean cupboard, helps me get rid of objects that are just taking up space. Although this process can be tedious and a bit painful, it feels wonderful to have identified and saved just what you want to continue having in your life. You know you don't have to dig through things in the cupboard that are no longer of any use. And you can see that space has been created for what comes next.

Take a moment to notice how the analogy of cupboard cleaning applies to your life and the career, education, and roles you had in the past.

MY TALENTS AND SKILLS

Now, return to the Chapter 1 Homework Assignment and take a look at the items on your "My Careers/Jobs" list.

Spend some time with each item (including the ones you have crossed out). Picture the talents/skills you mastered in that career, degree, or role.

In the area below, start a new list of these talents/skills, making note of your discoveries. This will be a good list to revisit as new awareness arises.

MY TALENTS/SKILLS

_____

_____

_____

_____

_____

_____

_____

_____

Now, let's take a look at any sense of loss you may be experiencing.

HAS THE VALUE OF YOUR PAST WORK DISAPPEARED?

It is not unusual to feel a sense of loss and emptiness at this time. Honor the grieving/loss you are feeling. *And* start to be aware of the space that is opening up for new adventures.

Know that this is an ongoing process of awareness; feel free to return to thinking on this subject and make a mental note of any new realizations that come to you.

> *If you want your life*
> *to be a magnificent story,*
> *then begin by realizing*
> *that you are the author.*
> —Mark Houlahan

Through this activity, you will find that your career and roles probably developed skills and capabilities you can use in other ways. For instance, if your job required you to speak to clients about a product your company manufactured, this skill can be turned into teaching or mentoring people who need help learning a new subject. In discovering the talents that are yours to keep, you are recognizing the value of what you did in the past. I like the analogy of preparing a garden for planting. For those of you who have done this, you know how important it is to remove all the weeds that are taking up space and may overtake the new plants that are beginning to grow. The exercise you are doing here will provide fertile ground in which to plant the seeds of your new life. As hard as it is to give up those treasured items, remember you are "preparing your garden." And, most important of all, now that all the weeds are gone, you have room to grow your new life.

HONOR THE SENSE OF LOSS YOU ARE FEELING

Some people will find letting go harder than others and see this as a process they just don't want to do. For them, moving into a perceived empty space is at best uncomfortable and at worst like denying all the hard work that got them to this point. These are the people who will often center their conversations on the past experiences in their lives. Their chats will include details about the careers they loved, the people they used to know, even the scores of their best golf games; you know, "The good old days." They don't relate to the future; they don't see themselves there yet. Of course, it's tempting to want to turn back to what was, like comfort food on a sorely trying day.

When you take off one set of clothes,
you are naked for a minute before you
put on another. When age is seen in a purely
material context, you sort of wonder if
there is another set of clothes.
—Marianne Williamson
The Gift of Change: Spiritual Guidance
for a Radically New life

Marianne Williamson describes this period of time as "living the in-between times." This is a perfect description of not being sure where you are or where you are going. During this period, you may experience feelings of longing and discontent. For many people, there is a grieving and mourning process that accompanies moving away from the known and comfortable past. Grief is, quite simply, part of the process of changing perception. By changing your perception, you change your relationship to your life from what it was to what it is to be. I encourage you to step forward into the feelings that arise. (We will be working on this in the homework section of this chapter.) It is important that you allow yourself to "feel what you are feeling" so that you can move through your fears and doubts, and on to what's next. Stay with these feelings for a while and ask yourself:

"What is this discomfort asking me to notice?"

Hint: As we continue, you will notice (if you haven't already) that your life is always speaking to you! And encouraging you to persevere and work through the discomfort.

Elizabeth Kubler-Ross has described grief and mourning in stages she observed while working with terminally ill patients and their loved ones. More recently, it has been observed that the same stages can be used to describe the feelings that accompany many significant life changes. I have edited these definitions to better fit the work we are doing here. Please recognize that the stages aren't linear. In our day-to-day lives, they don't occur neatly one after another. In all reality, they may occur in any order and, for you, possibly not at all. I am including this discussion here because I have identified these steps as happening in my own life during times of transition and change.

Denial — The first reaction is often denial. In this stage the individual believes they are not having a problem, that everything is just fine, or that the feelings they are having are not associated with the end of their career.

Anger — When the individual recognizes that denial cannot continue, they may become frustrated with themselves and with others. If this phase had a language, it might be saying, "What's wrong with me? I should be happy: I have all the time, money, etc., I need to do everything I want." Or, if their retirement was not their choice, "Why me? It's not fair! How can this happen to me? Who is to blame? How could I have prevented this from happening?"

Bargaining — The third stage involves the hope that the individual can talk himself or herself out of the feelings he or she is having. These individuals may look endlessly at ways they can find peace: "if I take better care of myself," "if I use this time to help others," "if I just went back to work."

Depression — During the fourth stage, the sadness and depression may make the individual feel hopeless. In this state, the individual may simply withdraw—"What's the use?"—and feel like any effort is too much.

Acceptance — This stage allows one to open up to new possibilities. "It's going to be OK. I can look objectively at my new life. Nothing is impossible." At this point, they can face future change and see a light at the end of the tunnel. They can look optimistically at what comes next, and have the courage to step into the new ideas and experiences that appear.

Remember, these feelings may occur for you, or they may not. They might occur from time to time. This description is presented to help you better understand the process you may be having and to realize it is just a way for you to work through and identify what you are experiencing.

Change your thoughts
and you change your world.
—Norman Vincent Peale

For me, this experience occurred when I was dealing with the issue of renewing my California state dental hygiene license. I worked many years to acquire this license and I renewed it several times after I had retired, even though I knew I was not going to work as a hygienist again. I couldn't help remembering the many freeway trips I took from Garden Grove to UCLA, usually at 6:15 a.m., often returning late at night. And I proudly remembered all I had learned and accomplished; it was truly a wonderful time for me. However, after five years, I eventually tired of amassing the continuing education units required and gave myself permission not to renew, to let the license go. It was time to be honest with myself and prepare for the future life I was moving into.

This can also be your opportunity to revisit your decision, your commitment to create a wonderful rest of your life. And, as you continue through this book, you will gather the tools needed to recommit to yourself.

Let's look at what **Gregg Braden**, author of *Resilience from the Heart: The Power to Thrive in Life's Extremes*, has to say about this period of life. He describes a transitional time as a period where it's important to be honest with yourself and prepare for change. This happens more readily if you positively center your thoughts on "pivoting into another role."

He describes several key points that are pertinent to your present process of self-exploration.

Be Honest With Yourself. Ask yourself how the world feels different at this time of your life. Embrace the fact that your life is changing in ways you hadn't anticipated. Take a look at what this means to you.

Identify Your Core Values. Ask yourself what your core value system has been based upon: Is it material wealth, personal well-being, spirituality/religion, self-esteem, self-importance, or a combination of these values? Your answers will give you clarity in navigating through this time of your life.

Examining and becoming clear about what you are feeling and defining your personal values allows you to acquire more self-knowledge. As you increase your personal insight and inner clarity, you will find you are better prepared to meet the challenges of your changing world.

I suggest that you spend some quiet time with the steps in this process. As you find your own answers, make notes in the lined area below. This will provide an area to continue this conversation with yourself as you progress.

NOTES FROM GREGG BRADEN QUOTE

_____

_____

_____

_____

_____

_____

_____

_____

_____

_____

Do you press the "pause" button –
the "until" button in life –
by saying "I can't be happy until...?"
Press the "play" button and rejoice
in the nowness of the moment.
—Michael Bernard Beckwith

A LITTLE EXERCISE FOR YOU

So, let's do a little exercise to demonstrate the power of "letting go." You may have seen it before, but it is a good demonstration of what we discussed above. Call this the Fist Exercise.

First, take your nondominant hand and make a tight fist.

Second, with your other hand, pry at the fingers of your closed fist as if trying to force it open.

You will discover you can't open your clenched fist! This is a good analogy for the strength you can use to hold onto the past.

Third, willingly open your clenched hand and shake your fingers. How were you able to do this?

You consciously used the power of your mind. The aspect of your mind that opened your hand can be used to open yourself and reach for the future.

What if ... Everything you're
going through right now
is preparing you for a dream
bigger than you can imagine?
—Renee A. Sauter

CONSIDER THE CONCEPT THAT SPACE IS BEING CREATED FOR "WHAT'S NEXT"

I discovered the statement, "If not now, when?" about the same time I decided not to renew my dental hygiene license. Hearing this statement provided a fascinating epiphany for me. It became my measuring stick to use when faced with the possibility of a new experience. What I discovered (and what many of the people I interviewed for this book discovered) was that there are many new experiences just waiting to be tried. What was I waiting for? It was all a matter of looking at this period of my life with an open mind. You can bet that, during this time, you will need to call on your courage. You may even feel a bit vulnerable.

You will discover there's a whole new reality out there and, just like a new dress/suit, it is waiting to be tried on. You may find that this new outfit doesn't fit you just right; but keep looking for what feels good! Keep your eyes and ears open! There's a whole world full of options, opportunities you would never find if you didn't try them on. It has been my experience that one good "outfit" leads to another. One interesting new person will lead to another interesting time for you. Guaranteed! Allow me to quote myself:

It is my experience,
when I decide to no longer do an activity,
I discover that something even more exciting
comes along to fill that space.
—Ginni Gordon

I also like the analogy of a rainy day. If you wake up to a downpour, you can respond in a couple of ways. You can say, "Oh no, it's raining. This whole day is ruined, and it's going to be difficult: difficult to get around, depressingly dark and cloudy, not fun at all." Or you could respond in another way. "Oh goody, it's raining! I can finish that book I started and get some of the things done around the house I have been wanting to do." Both decisions set the pace for the day. The day is the same, but the experience is totally different! I came to realize that, if I had faith that life was going to expose me to a smorgasbord of adventures, then I could approach each event, each day, like a kid on Christmas Eve, excitedly waiting to see what was in the presents under the tree.

Whenever you find yourself
doubting how far you can go,
just remember how far you have come.
Remember everything you have faced,
and all the battles you have won.
—Unknown

MARY ELLEN CARTER'S STORY

I met with my friend Mary Ellen Carter in her darling beach cottage in Laguna Beach. She had prepared a lovely tea, and our interview was an enjoyable experience for us both. She was an obvious choice for this chapter. I was able to see where she had taken her career skills and moved them into a totally different arena. During her working life she was a career counselor at several community colleges in Southern California: Golden West, Cypress, Fullerton, Rio Hondo and Irvine Valley. Her role had been to assist students in career and life planning and job development. A colleague was taking a sabbatical and asked that she take over her career classes full-time. This would have cut into the trips Mary Ellen had planned with her husband, so she declined. Mary Ellen's husband, David Carter, is a federal district judge. He travels to other countries and does judiciary training and presides over international court cases.

Mary Ellen was invited by the government of Malawi, Africa, to accompany her husband, who was going to lecture to a conference of the Supreme Court justices in the area. She loved the trip and everything about Africa. And that was where her dream was revealed. She discovered where to apply her expertise: using education to change lives. That is how Direct Connections to Africa began.

In this area of Malawi, high school students need to pay for their education, and many are forced to quit because of lack of funds. While in Malawi, Mary Ellen traveled to different high schools in the district and selected good students who didn't have the money to pay their school fees. When she returned to the United States, she held small get-togethers, asking people to sponsor a student or a teacher so they could continue to attend school. The students were also required to give back. As a counselor, Mary Ellen believes that helping people is meeting them halfway. The sponsored students and teachers were required to give back by writing monthly letters and keeping their sponsors updated on their progress and their life in Malawi. When I met Mary Ellen, she had secured sponsors for the eligible students she had selected, so I sponsored a teacher. I sent him a box every month or two containing school supplies and used textbooks donated by my daughter, who taught the same subjects here in the United States.

The village was located in an area that had no source of running water. The water had to be carried from the river, and girls were designated to do this chore. Because the water was not pure (it had a yellow-green color), many of the children had intermittent, water-related illnesses, some of them quite serious. In America, we take having pure water for granted; but in Malawi, it wasn't even available. I could not shake the image of the young girls whose lives were consumed by the 10-mile round trip carrying water—and bad water at that.

When my dad passed away in 2013, he left me a small inheritance. The idea for a well in this village popped into my head, and I asked Mary Ellen to find out whether building a well would be possible. The answer was an enthusiastic yes, and the six-month process of construction took place. The well has a bench around the pump where the women can sit and talk as they wait their turn. I can feel my dad smiling down on these women as they gather the pure water. And I can happily add that waterborne illnesses have dropped dramatically and that the children of the village are healthier. Since this time, donations have added more wells. There are now nine wells in surrounding villages. Mary Ellen has appointed four representatives to organize the wells, two men and two women. Before a village can get a well, a committee needs to be formed to take care of the proposed well, and her representatives take care of this process.

Over the last eight years, the program has continued to develop. It now includes tuition for high school and college students. One student I sponsored in the last few years has graduated from college and is now an accountant for the water district. It is very rewarding to watch a student learn and grow, and get a job that changes their life.

Direct Connections to Africa now provides preschool buildings, teacher connections, recreation, and high school and college scholarships. Mary Ellen has just started a job-development placement program because many people in third-world countries don't know what to do with their education. Several of the more recent additions are bikes for people starting businesses, sewing machines to promote the manufacturing of items for sale, and ambulance bikes to transport patients who are at a distance from health care.

Mary Ellen Carter is a wonderful example of what can happen if you keep your eyes open to possibilities. You never know when an opportunity will arise and what adventures are awaiting you when you take a risk, when you try something a little different and say "yes" to life.

The quotation that follows is from a woman whose life's work has touched millions of hearts. She said "yes" to life.

Stay afraid, but do it anyway.
What's important is the action.
You don't have to wait to be confident.
Just do it and eventually
the confidence will follow
—Carrie Fisher
1956 – 2016

HOMEWORK ASSIGNMENT – CHAPTER 2

This has been a busy chapter. Let's review some of the work you have done up to now.

1. You looked again at your list My Careers/Jobs that you began in the Chapter 1 Homework Assignment.
2. You are now going to spend some time with each career and role, honoring the memories, the feelings of pride, of grief, and loss of identity that may arise.

While evaluating each item, we will use a short exercise I call *Pause And Picture This*. It will assist you in getting in touch with how you are feeling. It goes like this:

First, bring to mind one of the careers/jobs you have had and will be evaluating.

Next, ask yourself these questions:

- "How do I picture myself and what sense of myself do I have while in this career/job?"
- "What am I thinking and feeling right now about saying goodbye (or having said goodbye, if it's a former job) to this part of my life?"

Using the lined area on the next page, list the career/role from your original list and add the feelings you have identified in the *Pause And Picture This* exercise.

CAREER/ROLE FEELINGS

_____

_____

_____

_____

_____

_____

_____

_____

_____

_____

_____

_____

3. Now, using the lined area on the next page, start a new dialogue with yourself, asking this question:

"What are some areas that might open up for new exploration/expression within the newfound freedom of my retirement?"

This can be an ongoing conversation with yourself. Use your imagination (even more than your logic) and realize that creativity will help you with this exercise.

NEW AREAS FOR EXPLORATION/EXPRESSION

_____

_____

_____

_____

_____

_____

_____

_____

_____

_____

_____

4. Examine the items on the list of "Talents And Skills" you created earlier in this chapter, and place a star by the ones that feel the most significant at this time. Think of these items as valuable tools you are taking forward into your new life.

In the area provided on the next page, list these important items. Spend some time with this task, generously adding any additional skills that come to mind.

MY IMPORTANT TALENTS AND SKILLS

_____

_____

_____

_____

_____

_____

_____

_____

_____

_____

_____

_____

_____

_____

_____

_____

_____

_____

ADDITIONAL NOTES

_____

_____

_____

_____

_____

_____

_____

_____

_____

_____

_____

_____

_____

_____

_____

_____

_____

_____

CHAPTER 3
WHAT HAVE I BEEN TELLING ME ... ABOUT ME?

Initiate a habit of choosing
thoughts and ideas that
support feeling good and powerful,
and that elevate you to a
higher level of consciousness.
—Wayne Dyer

WATCH THE IDEAS THAT APPEAR RIGHT ABOUT NOW

Because it is important to be aware of what's happening in the arena of your thoughts, we are going to spend some concentrated time working on self-talk. Right about now, you may notice that you are experiencing "self-defeating" thoughts, thoughts that can make you feel this whole process is "just too much work" and "I have been through all this before; do I want/need to do this again?" It's true that you have worked diligently to create your life up to now. That tenacity is what is leading you to the adventure of designing the wonderful rest of your life.

I have discovered the value of confronting these negative ideas as they arise and "reframing" them into statements that are encouraging. I am sure you can see the benefit you will derive from this process. We will be working on making this a habit later in this chapter.

Another factor to take into consideration during the "reframing process" is explained by Anne Perrah, Ph.D., in her book, *Taken to Heart: Parenting Our Children and Re-Parenting Ourselves Through the Healing Power of Story*. Her principle goes like this: The Principle of Meaning-Making says, "There is what happens, and there is what we make it mean. Every time!" As you examine each belief, especially if it evokes a message that is self-defeating, take a look at the possibility of an underlying judgment and where it might have originated. For instance, it is possible to ascribe a meaning to an event that is not promoting your moving forward to the next part of your life. Perrah states further that with "time and experience, you can change what you remembered, how you remembered it, and thereby, change what you make it mean."

That "no" voice inside you
belongs to a grown-up
who was training you
to be scared—
a parent, a teacher,
an older sibling.
You have taken their
voice inside you and that's what's stopping you.
—Barbara Sher

I was invited to join the cast of a musical, "100 Years on Broadway," to provide the dancing needed for a few of the numbers. Everyone in the cast (including me) had a singing role of some kind, and I was intimidated by the beautiful voices I heard (one of our cast members sang "The Star-Spangled Banner" to open ball games). My initial self-statements were something like this: "Who are you kidding? You are going to just look plain ridiculous. Maybe you can stick to group songs . . ." The meaning I gave to the invitation was, "They only want me in the cast because I can dance." My inner critic was hard at work.

I decided that, rather than listen to this negative voice, I would take on the work of developing my voice. Luckily I found two wonderful teachers/friends who held my hand and taught me how to use my "instrument." Months later, when I was chatting with the director, she told me they asked me to be in the musical because they liked how I dedicated myself to parts I was given, and they liked my on-stage personality. As I continue to train and develop my voice, I am more comfortable with the songs I am given to sing. None of this could have happened if I hadn't confronted the negative ideas my inner critic was handing out.

As I said, the biggest challenge was in changing my attitude. I needed to let myself be a beginner and give myself credit for the progress I made along the way. And I had to stop comparing myself to the other cast members.

Almost every successful person
begins with two beliefs . . .
The future can be better
than the present,
and I have the power
to make it so.
—David Brooks

Most recently we have presented musicals based on the music of Irving Berlin and another featuring songs from movies. I now have confidence in my ability to use my voice, and I work steadily on learning the songs I am asked to sing. Once again, I saw that what my dad always told me was true: "You can accomplish anything if you want it bad enough and try hard enough."

> *The curious paradox is*
> *that when I accept myself*
> *just as I am,*
> *then I can change.*
> —Carl Rogers

CLEANING UP MY SELF-TALK, EXAMINING MY EXCUSES

Most of us have "internal conversations" with ourselves in which we are not always kind. Many of these thoughts go unnoticed but do affect how we see ourselves and how we measure our potential to move forward in our lives. Examining this self-talk can provide a wealth of information and allow us to take our foot off the brakes that may be slowing us down. The Carl Rogers quote is a gentle reminder of the power of self-acceptance.

So now let's gently begin working on the thoughts that you are telling you about you.

Find an additional notebook you can use specifically for this process. You can call it your Self-talk Notebook. I have found that writing these thoughts down makes them more manageable. Instead of feeling them swimming around in your consciousness, they become more definitive in black and white.

This process will be a little different because you will be writing a monologue concerning your unwanted feelings, ideas, and the self-judgments that are coming up and not serving you. I encourage you to use any language you want (even four-letter words, if that's what you are feeling). I have heard this called "throwing up on the page." And it can be just that cathartic. Remember, this is for your eyes only. So go for it. Write your list!

You will use this list in the homework assignment at the end of this chapter. And when you have finished using this list, I suggest you take this page and run it through the shredder or burn it. This is a symbolic way to discard these unwanted judgments and feelings. Keep this exercise in mind to use when unwanted thoughts appear.

Every day is an opportunity for a new life.
Every day you stand at the tipping point of your life.
And, on any one day,
you can change the future—
through the way that you feel.
—Rhonda Byrne

WHAT I WANT TO BE FEELING AND DOING RIGHT NOW

This is the perfect segue to taking a look at what you are feeling. If you had the choice, what would you like to be feeling right now? Use your imagination. What feelings would you rather be experiencing? I love this quote, often attributed to Abraham Lincoln. "People are usually about as happy as they decide to be." So examine the element of choice; we can *choose* to move forward through our angst and into an area where our natural enthusiasm takes over.

Before you retired, your life may have seemed as if you were in a comfortable existence inside a seashell; your fit was perfect and life was, for the most part, predictable. Now you have reached a place where you have outgrown your shell; you have been thrown into a new landscape, one in which the unfamiliar hills and valleys present a whole new way of moving through life. This can be both scary and exciting.

A good habit to adopt right now is to continue to watch your self-talk. If you discover you are thinking defeating thoughts, consciously replace them with positive ones. You can also call on the process you used earlier in this chapter: write them down in your Self-talk Notebook and discard them. This takes consistent effort, but it is worthwhile and has proved beneficial in my life.

Let's revisit the question we touched on in Chapter 1. It's an important question and an idea to acknowledge.

"HAVE I ALREADY DONE WHAT I SET OUT TO DO IN LIFE?"

It may be hard to move forward, to see a future, if you see all your goals as having been accomplished.

Recognize that this time of life will require that you be open to the new possibilities that present themselves.

Take some time with each opportunity that appears. Don't let yourself jump immediately into thinking "That's not for me" or "Oh, I wouldn't like that" without trying out this new experience. If you find you are feeling a sense of boredom or discouragement, get out your Self-talk Notebook and explore/discard what is standing in your way.

As you continue to do this work, you will discover that it helps you put into place methods/practices that will work for you. I have suggested some above and wanted to include excerpts of an article on luck written by Kathleen McCleary that appeared alongside an interview of Tom Brokaw, published in *Parade* magazine (May 3, 2015). McCleary discusses being open to change and watching for opportunities.

In the interview, Tom Brokaw discussed how others consider him to be lucky. He relates that, while he knows some experiences in life cannot be controlled, "A big part of making your own luck is just charging out of the gate every morning." Dr. Stephann Makri, a researcher of serendipity at City University London, says that if you "have your eyes open, recognize the unexpected when it occurs and take action," a sort of serendipity happens, seen by some as "luck." McCleary advises that we should open ourselves to these moments and watch what happens. She lays out a method, presented here in these steps, which I have shortened and made relevant to your taking your first steps into your new adventure.

1. **Pay Attention** – Curiosity, flexibility, courage and diligence are the traits that prepare you to recognize opportunities and act on them. Put down your cell phone, step away from your computer and television, look around and *listen*.

2. **Open Your Calendar** – You can be so busy that you miss the opportunity when it appears. Planning "down time" – walking, meditating, etc. – will allow new ideas to reveal themselves.

3. **Increase Your Odds** – If you sample more experiences, more possibilities will appear (this is where making notes in your soon-to-be-developed bucket list will come in handy). Occasionally, all I learned is "that's not for me," but this is valuable information. If you wait to take chances only when you're sure of success, you could miss out on some wonderful experiences.

4. **Take Chances** – New possibilities will more often occur if you take risks or go outside your comfort zone. Exposing yourself to new people, activities, places and information gives you the chance to make connections you had never imagined.

DENNIS McCARTER'S STORY

I'd like to introduce you to Dennis, whom I have dubbed the "non-retired retiree." We met for the interview at a Starbucks in Irvine, California, and settled in for a friendly conversation. I had known Dennis for a while, but this interview gave me a chance to really meet the man.

Dennis leaned forward across the table, looked me in the eye and said, "I'll never retire. I knew from the start that my talents were in the area of consulting, and I loved being part of the process." With a bachelor's degree in English literature and an MBA, he took his people management skills into well-recognized companies like Winchell's Donuts and the Denny's restaurant chain. They were so impressed with him that they offered him a job as president of Winchell's Donut House, Inc. He turned down the job, realizing he would ultimately be bored.

Over the years he handled major projects, including the massive effort of reorganizing the Irvine Company. Playing full-out has presented a few obstacles, including three financial downswings. "This comes with being a risk taker," he said. He's happy to report that he's doing well now.

At the age of 71, he took his time and talents in a new direction. He now assists nonprofit organizations in raising funds, a skill that can be difficult for some groups to manage. His company uses a process that takes much of the time and hassle out of this part of running a nonprofit and allows the group to focus their efforts on the goals they wish to accomplish.

His ability to define and direct this activity is a blessing to all of his clients.

START YOUR BUCKET LIST!

OK, now it's time to begin a Bucket List. You may or may not have done this before or, like me, you have thought about it but not gotten around to doing it. Or maybe these ideas have just been floating around in your head. This will be an enjoyable undertaking, one designed to encourage you to "color outside the lines." Make it a fun experience; you could even include items or actions you have dreamed of or started before for encouragement.

Mary Morrissey [see resource list], author, life coach and motivational speaker, suggests you use this question as a measuring device for this exercise:

> *What would I love to do if money,*
> *education, experience, gender,*
> *age and time were not factors*
> *to be considered and dealt with?*

Think about this statement:

"I have all the money, education, experience, gender, age and time I need."

What experience would I attempt if my "logical mind" wasn't busy telling me that I'm too old, I don't have enough money, I am not strong enough, etc.? What would I love to start to do/do next?

MY BUCKET LIST

Remember your criteria:

"I have all the money, education, experience, gender, age and time I need."

_____

_____

_____

_____

_____

_____

_____

_____

_____

_____

_____

_____

As you work on this list, be aware that this is just a departure point. The fact that you have this ongoing list means you can put in additions as they come to your mind. I have benefited many times from beginning a list, placing it on a counter in the kitchen, and running to make additional notes as thoughts came to me. And, believe me, when you start this list, ideas will come to mind. This is the luck that Tom Brokaw mentioned. This also works on the computer: start a list and watch to see what appears. Writing this book has been an exercise for me in using this tool.

Your Bucket List can be the soil in which to grow something new. Just let yourself plant the seeds of what you would find enjoyable to do, and watch the seedlings grow. The items you list might not turn out to be the right ones for you, but they could lead to another experience you would enjoy. When you examine an item you have included and decide it probably would not be a good fit, determine what it is that lights you up about the prospect of this experience. Have a good time with this and consider the possibility of including any service or mentor work that appeals to you.

If you feel the need for further inspiration (or just want to explore other possibilities), I have listed two books in the Book List in the back of this book that provide food for thought.

The books are: *I Could Do Anything If I Only Knew What It Was* by **Barbara Sher** and *65 Things to Do When You Retire,* edited by **Mark Evan Chimsky**.

Of course, we all have a mental [bucket] list
of things we'd like to do, once we retire.
. . . rather than being driven by what you've been missing,
it's more powerful to intentionally identify
all the elements you truly desire,
which will support your well-being.
—From a chapter by John E. Nelson, in the book
65 Things to Do When You Retire

HOMEWORK ASSIGNMENT – CHAPTER 3

Now, reexamine the items in the list you made in your Self-talk Notebook.
On the next page, let your logical mind take over and rewrite each statement in a positive way, turning these negative thoughts into positive ones.

Take each statement individually and reframe each phrase. For instance, ideas like "I'm too old to. . ." may be replaced with thoughts like "I now have all the time I need to learn. . ."

As you look at each thought, add positive encouragement for yourself as a sort of internal "Pep Talk." Speak to yourself as if you were counseling a good friend. What would you say to this person if he or she were facing the same feelings you are having?

Be sure to include the qualities about yourself you find worthwhile and commendable (remember, you are seeing yourself through a friend's eyes).

Give this activity quality time; it provides powerful insight and awareness of who you are and what you are capable of doing/becoming. This also provides a good place to identify the meaning and the feelings as they arise and restate them. Develop this practice into a wonderful habit for yourself. It can truly change your perspective of yourself. It's as simple as saying "no" to these thoughts when you see them appear; then decide to change what you are thinking to a positive statement. You can destroy the list from your Self-talk Notebook when you are done with this assignment.

MY PEP TALK

Extra Credit Exercise: This is what I call a "Mirror Exercise." Read the encouraging items on the above list aloud to yourself in front of a mirror (even if it feels a little silly or uncomfortable). This can be a very powerful way to plant these new concepts in your mind.

CHAPTER 4

WHAT YOU NEED NOW IS COURAGE, INTUITION, AND COMMITMENT

Fear is both a challenge and an opportunity
because it signals our minds that
a change is trying to emerge.
—Dr. Jim Turrell

BE WILLING TO BE A BEGINNER . . . AGAIN, AND TRY ON A NEW HAT

You are now entering a place of being a beginner . . . again. Is there a resistance inside saying, "Oh no, not this again?" This time can be kind of like the first day of first grade. Do you have any memories of that experience? Or was it the first day of a new job that made you think, "I am not sure I'm ready for this."

Hugh Laurie, star of the TV show *House,* puts it well. "It is a terrible thing, I think, in life, to wait until you are ready. I have this feeling now that actually no one is ever ready to do anything. There is almost no such thing as ready. There is only now. And you may as well do it now. Generally speaking, now is as good a time as any."

In January 2010, a meeting at The Center for Spiritual Living focused on a new play that was in the works. It was to be about historical women and their contributions to the rights we ladies enjoy in the present day. I attended, thinking I could contribute to any dance scenes that might be included. I wanted to be part of this group; I really enjoyed the air of creativity circulating in that room and the aliveness of the women there.

Everyone who attended was required to read one of the parts. I picked the part of Mary Kay Ash. Honestly? Because it had the fewest lines!

The director called me later that day and told me, "You got the part." *I got the part?* I'm not an actress; I had never acted a day in my life. After some thought, however, I decided "What the heck?" and gave it a try.

The part of me that was fairly new at "coloring outside the lines" was asking "Egad, what's she getting us into?" During rehearsals, the kind and wonderful director guided my shaky, new actress legs through the beginning runthroughs. I put on my "big girl panties" and let the wonder of the stage take hold of me.

The play is called *We Did It For You*, by Thea Iberall, and we have performed it at many different venues for many different audiences. In addition to Mary Kay Ash, I now play Eleanor Roosevelt and Billie Jean King. So much fun!

Apprehension and fear are like mountains; once you master climbing them, you will discover you have learned new skills that will serve you when you reach the next crest. If you find yourself feeling apprehensive—a little (or a lot) scared—take a moment. Consider the possibility that under the uneasiness you are experiencing is an excitement and enthusiasm for "what's next." Now is when you can call on the courage and stamina you have developed over the years to assist you.

We were born to be free,
to expand our horizons
by going where we have never gone before,
and not hang out in the relative comfort
and safety of the nest, the known.
There is a place within us that is
courageous beyond our
human understanding;
it yearns to explore
beyond the boundaries
of our daily life.
—Dennis Merritt Jones
The Art of Uncertainty:
How to Live in the Mystery of Life and Love It

BE WILLING TO BE VULNERABLE. YOU'RE LEARNING A NEW GAME TO PLAY

Now is the time to allow yourself to be vulnerable, and that's not easy. You have spent many years becoming accomplished in many areas, and now life is asking you to begin again. Do you feel the bile rising in your throat, creating a sense of nausea? Are your armpits getting damp as you hope your deodorant is still working? Are you tempted to settle for the easy chair in front of the TV and watch reruns?

If you think you can, or
if you think you can't,
you're right!
—Henry Ford

David Whyte puts it this way,

"Whenever we attempt something difficult
there is always a sense that we have to wake
some giant slumbering inside ourselves,
some greater force as yet hidden from us.
We need to stir this inner giant to life
in order to find the strength
to live out the life we want for ourselves."

A NEW GAME PLAN?

Why not approach this season of your life like you would if you were training to play a new game? Call it a "learning experience." You've been a beginner before, and you can do it again. Even though this may seem difficult, it's time to encourage yourself just like you would encourage a friend starting out on a new path.

Anne Perrah describes this period as "having a case of the 'overwhelms.'" It's that point in our life when change—and change we have freely chosen and truly want—reaches that state of complexity where we cannot decide what to do next.

Forward progress can grind to a standstill and our energy, like a housebound puppy, seems to be chasing its own tail. A friend of mine once offered me a strategy for overcoming the disabling effects of the "overwhelms." One way of getting a sense of this helpful tool is to revisit your "beginner's mind," to lighten up and become "as a little child."

Anne describes a process that she learned in her spiritual psychology program at University of Santa Monica. Let's imagine for a moment you are that little child, and someone's goal is to teach you how to successfully throw a beanbag into a bucket. First, see yourself guided to stand very near the bucket and just get a feel for releasing the beanbag. Next, you would be introduced to the challenge of the toss from a little distance. You are successful, and you feel elated! After the positive reinforcement of a few three-foot tosses, feeling quite successful, you are challenged to move farther back. You soon discover that farther back the toss is not as easy to accomplish successfully. But you had those three-foot tosses down to maximum success!

For our purposes, let's leave the child there, and translate this mental exercise into a tool for you to create maximum forward motion and positive action toward realizing your personal goal. When confronted with the discouragement and frustration of the "overwhelms," just imagine the sense of relief and pleasure you derive from chunking down to size a series of deliberate, manageable, "three-foot tosses." See yourself moving steadily forward again, and your process of change will be back on track!

As you step out onto this new road, remember: no one expects to walk onto the soccer field and kick a perfect goal the first time. It takes many hours of practice to get that ball to go where you want it to go. This period of your life will respond to you being patient and supportive of yourself.

Occasionally, you will try something that turns out to be "not your cup of tea." But you will have learned something. You found something you can cross off your list as a possible new adventure. And you can give yourself credit for making the effort. In my experience, it becomes easier each time.

I remember the first time we performed our play, *We Did It For You*, and I stepped onto the stage as Mary Kay Ash, wearing a bright pink jacket, rhinestone jewelry, and lots of makeup. I knew my lines, had developed a somewhat believable Texas accent, and was determined to do my best. It was an awesome experience that became easier with each performance.

BE WILLING TO LISTEN TO YOUR INTUITION

Using your intuition is a process that, once developed, will be handy in many areas of your life. You have amassed much wisdom over the years, and your intuition helps you put this wisdom into inspired action. This is a muscle that, when exercised, will serve you well. **Mary Morrissey** (*No Less Than Greatness*) describes it this way: "I have found that we have a divine side in us that knows what we must do. I also know that we have a very human nature that is less confident." As you exercise your intuition muscle, you reassure the part of you that needs your loving support to move forward along your path.

First: To aid you in recognizing and developing this ability, it helps to ask yourself a question that will tap into this skill. The clearer the question, the more you will be able to utilize the answer.

One of my favorite beginning questions is:

"What do I want?"

Another question I find helpful is:

"What is important to me right now?"

Or, to put what you want in another way:

"What is my dream for the next part of my life?"

Continue to formulate questions, bringing in your creativity to help exercise this "intuition muscle." List your questions below:

QUESTIONS FROM MY INTUITION

_____

_____

_____

_____

_____

_____

_____

_____

_____

_____

_____

Next, keeping each individual question in mind, sit quietly and examine the ideas that are bubbling to the surface.

Ask yourself the question out loud. Then sit quietly again and listen to what your "still, small voice" has to tell you. Experiment with this process; it is well worth the time.

Listening to your intuition is a skill that serves you in many ways. Some people report that they feel their intuition in the pit of their stomach—a gut feeling. Whatever form your intuition takes, it is a handy way to stay in touch with what your inner wisdom has to tell you. At this period of your life, you have so much left to experience and so many tools to help you discover where you want to go.

I recently saw, on my computer, an excerpt of an interview with Steven Spielberg in which he was discussing this very thing—listening for a dream. He relates it like this: "When your dream speaks to you, it doesn't come at you screaming in your face. It always whispers; it never shouts. And if you can listen to the whisper, and what it says 'tickles your heart,' it is what you are to do. And you and the rest of the world will benefit from this."

Have you ever listened to someone who talks very quietly? You usually have to listen carefully to understand the message he or she is telling you. That "still, small voice" that has guided you to many accomplishments in the past is still there. It's like having your own internal compass, one that will always point to "true north," toward what is your best and highest good.

As you continue using this exercise, you will grow in your ability to trust the route your "inner knower" is telling you to take. Spend some time with this exercise; use the space on the following page to develop and write down your impressions. This is a good time to give up any "right" or "wrong" concerns. Make this a fun experiment.

ANSWERS FROM MY INTUITION

_____

_____

_____

_____

_____

_____

_____

_____

_____

_____

_____

_____

_____

_____

_____

_____

_____

_____

_____

_____

The last step is to put the messages you are receiving into operation. My experience tells me that if I want my intuition to stay in contact with me, I need to pay attention *and* act. **Dennis Merritt Jones** puts it this way:

"Every time you have a choice to make
and you don't make it, by default,
you are making a choice not to make a choice, which is, of course, a choice . . .
the more conscious you are about your choices,
the more likely it is you will end up
where you want to be
at the end of your stay on this planet."

As you begin working on this part of the exercise, you may find it helpful to ask yourself,

"What can I do today that will move me in the direction I want to go?"

I often find it helpful to make notes about the impressions I am receiving. It has also been my experience that as I am making these notes, more of the message appears. Remember, this is your process; use it in a way that works effectively for you. Practice and experiment a little until you find what "feels right," and know you are developing a valuable new tool.

Ask yourself what is really important
and then have the wisdom and courage
to build your life around your answer.
—Unknown

Record here what "yourself" answered:

_____

_____

_____

_____

_____

_____

_____

_____

_____

_____

_____

_____

_____

_____

_____

_____

_____

LOOK FOR HELP/SUPPORT.
FIND NEW TEACHERS/HEROES

Whenever you find yourself doubting how far you can go,
just remember how far
you have come.
Remember everything you have faced, all the battles you have won,
and all the fears you have overcome.
—Unknown

As you continue the process of change, you may find it valuable to reach out for help and support. A good friend or a person who has been through the retiring/*refire*-ing process can tune into your frustration and your feelings of vulnerability. He or she can reassure you and remind you of how you succeeded in the past. Friends can also help you have "curiosity conversations" like "What do I want to do with the rest of my life?" Or they can help you with some of the intuitive questions you are working on.

Use the concept of the compass again. This person can act as your compass. You are starting out in a new direction. Your compass/friend can help you find your way through this unfamiliar terrain. He or she can be your guide by keeping you heading true north. I found it helpful to have a friend keep asking me:

"What do you want right now?"

"What is important to you right now?"

"What do you see as a possible first step?"

I also discovered that finding a way to accomplish that "first step" will prepare you for when the "next step" is ready to reveal itself. We will do further work on "first steps" in a future chapter.

You will find, as you move along this path, that more opportunities for new experiences will appear. Each time I tried something new, like acting in the play about historical women, I met someone who offered me another opportunity to flap my wings. When I first retired, I could not have even begun to describe the life I am leading today.

When I took my teaching classes at California State College, Long Beach, one of my professors made this statement: "Success breeds success." He was referring to giving your students a chance to succeed, but the saying applies nicely right here, in the retirement arena. Each step reveals another chance to find and develop the new you.

I visit a coffee shop in my neighborhood at that time in the morning when my energy is starting to wane. I often see the same group of guys sitting, drinking coffee, and having their "Starbucks Experience." Their conversation always looks animated; I'm sure they're solving the problems of the world. The point is that they are enjoying themselves and each other. And, I'll bet, enjoying having the time to just sit and share their life experiences.

DR. PAULINE MERRY'S STORY

Pauli Merry and I met when we were part of the cast of *We Did It For You*. We both played multiple roles: she played Sojourner Truth, the Reverend Pauli Murray, and Rosa Parks. As I mentioned, I was Eleanor Roosevelt, Mary Kay Ash and Billie Jean King. When it was time to look for people to interview, Pauli came to mind.

She described her last job, provost of the Pacific Coast Campus of Long Beach City College, as the best job she ever had. She was hired as an administrative dean, the only administrator on the oft-ignored smaller campus of the college, where most of the students were non-white and older than those on the larger campus. She made such an impact there that she was promoted to vice president, and then to provost.

Sadly, this idyllic job took a sharp turn in her final year there. The school's president retired. Pauli applied to be her replacement, not realizing that her successor had already been chosen. At this point, various actions were taken to make her life difficult enough that she would quit. She hung in there, but it was miserable for her. After the new president was in office, he told her that once her resignation letter was on his desk, her life would once again be wonderful. She gave him the letter and her life was very nice . . . until her forced retirement began.

Retirement for her was, at first, very difficult. She had been forced out of her dream job and now had to figure out what she would do with all of her talent, wisdom, and energy for the rest of her life. It took her a good decade to work out an answer she could live with.

I asked Pauli if she had any advice for people retiring—whether they are being forced out or are retiring by choice. In her case, she said she should have taken charge of the situation as much as possible (to keep from feeling like a victim). She recommended talking to the people in charge and stating your truth about what you see going on. Had she done this, she believes, it would have helped her come to an understanding of the whole process. Then she could have taken steps—not necessarily to keep her position, but to have a sense of personal control.

She is convinced it is imperative that a person have plans for "what's next." While the financial aspects of retirement are important, she told me, she feels it is even more important to have plans that fulfill the social and psychological void that often occurs when one retires. Having these plans is particularly important for people whose careers, like hers, were intensely interactive and highly interpersonal.

What is Pauli doing now after almost 10 years of retirement? She has finally completed the mourning period of leaving her dream job and has moved on, accepting new things that come along with a renewed sense of purpose and optimism. Such things include remaining active with friends, going to the theater, tutoring, giving dinner parties, and volunteering. The most unusual thing she has done is declare herself a music major at a college she once served as a vice president. Pauli is sharpening her skills as a cellist, going to classes and playing in community orchestras and small groups. She fancies herself one day as a jazz cellist ready to play at your next party.

HOMEWORK ASSIGNMENT CHAPTER 4

In this assignment, we are going to expand on the work you have done in this chapter. First, ask yourself:

What do I want right now?

What is important to me right now?

What do I see as a possible first step?

Next: Spend a few minutes listening to your intuition, making notes of the idea/ideas that occur to you on the following lines. Remember, you don't have to have a concrete goal for this exercise, only an inkling of a possibility. You can return to this page when new ideas come to you.

MY IDEAS/IMPRESSIONS

_____

_____

_____

_____

_____

_____

_____

_____

_____

_____

_____

_____

CHAPTER 5
"SHOW ME DA MONEY!"

Money is a means to an end,
not the end itself.
You cannot eat money,
and it cannot keep you warm
or cuddle you at night.
. . . the goal [of having money]
is to use it to do
whatever your heart
leads you to do,
and to do that which fulfills
your divine purpose.
—Edwene Gaines

DO I NEED MORE MONEY FOR THIS PERIOD OF MY LIFE?

Take a moment to remember the puzzle pieces life presented to you when you began thinking of retiring. Which pieces/experiences did you need to put into place before you were confident about the picture you saw? Are you still working on this puzzle? Are your finances one of those pieces? Do any of these thoughts generate a sense of fear? If so, know that you are not alone. As **Edwene Gaines** *(The Four Spiritual Laws of Prosperity: A Simple Guide to Unlimited Abundance)* says,

"Start thinking about some of the things that frighten you—especially those things that you would really love to do, that you have dreamed of doing, but that you were too fearful to do."

You may find that, although you have reached a place where you want to retire, you are not sure you have enough put aside to last you for the rest of your life. Many factors come into play at this point, including the rising cost of living, possible future health expenses, and the "big unknown". . . how many more years do I really need to provide for? This may be a good time to reassure yourself, or for **Deepak Chopra** *(Creating Affluence: The A-to-Z Steps to a Richer Life)* to reassure you with these words:

"Wealth consciousness is so much more
than having the ability to make money.
It's a mind-set that involves seeing life,
not as a struggle, but as a magical adventure
where our needs are met with grace and ease."

I made the choice to hire a financial planner; he had all the charts, graphs, and figures I needed to take into consideration to formulate my decision. He has continued to be a wonderful source of management and support for me.

There are many organizations offering help to make decisions in this area. What is essential is to remember that the "wealth consciousness" that Chopra describes is a state of mind. It's really knowing that what we need in our life is available to us. If you do your research knowing that what you need is available, you will find the company/person to guide you through the decisions you need to make.

You might decide to continue earning some money to cushion what you have saved. This is a good time to look creatively at how that can happen. Be aware that the need for extra money can also arise in ways you haven't planned.

AL HICKS' STORY

Let me introduce you to Al. He is a good friend I met when I became Ms. Senior Orange County. He has a beautiful speaking voice and is called on to be the emcee of many of our shows. We decided to have the interview over a steak at Outback Steakhouse.

This is his story: Al began his business career early in life, managing a multimillion-dollar jewelry business before he graduated from junior college. During his career, he obtained a gemology degree, trained business and sales managers, and ran small businesses, including a group of RadioShacks.

He retired at age 62; he and his wife traveled for much of the next eight years. Al was 69 when he and his wife divorced, and he found himself experiencing a major life change. He moved to a manufactured home community (in his words, "not a trailer park"), and realized he was going to need more income to meet his future needs. The lady who sold him his home suggested he join the onsite sales team.

So he studied the field of home sales, got his license, and went to work. He presents homes mainly in the park in which he lives, which is convenient. He keeps an eye out for new listings while he walks his dog. The job makes him feel "energized," and he enjoys working.

His sales skills transferred nicely to this new (to him) field, and he is doing well financially. To quote Al, "A competent salesperson can sell any product/service as long as they have knowledge of what they represent and good guidance to begin with." He has reached the point where his caring personality brings him referrals, and he is doing well.

During this time of change, he met and joined two performance groups and developed friendships with people who, he feels, enrich his life. These performance groups allow him to utilize his performance and presentation skills, and add greatly to the finished delivery of the shows.

He particularly enjoys doing shows for those who cannot get out to attend them (many of the shows take place at assisted living facilities) and for veterans, to honor their service to our country.

Al is also a longtime, active member of the National Exchange Club. This organization presents events that serve all areas of the community, from youth to police recognition.

SINGLE, DIVORCED, WIDOWED, ETC.

When you retire and you are living alone, you often face retirement issues from a different perspective. Decisions that a couple make together often draw on their individual and combined strengths. As a single person, you need to be "all the parts" or, as I like to say, "the buck stops here." For many retirees, there is a reduction in their income, and, although you may have done some/much planning for this time, you will probably face financial decisions that are, at best, challenging.

When I retired, I had been a widow for almost ten years. My husband died at an early age, so I had dealt with many of the concerns that arise for people when they find their life changing and they are alone. I had faced seeing my income reduced (pretty drastically) and had a competent financial advisor in place. I also had the issue of affordable housing already taken care of. I have watched others faced with this prospect deal with it in other ways, some of them very creatively.

For instance, one woman and her daughter decided to sell their respective homes and buy a larger home together. This was a good financial decision for them both.

One thing I did need to establish was a support system and contact with other people. In my experience, when you are alone, you face additional stress factors that are made easier by reaching out for help. Upon retirement, I knew I needed assistance to manage my finances, but I also realized I needed help dealing with many of the concerns I had previously discussed with my coworkers.

When your work friends are no longer around, it is more of an effort to get the feedback you may need. Sure, you can probably figure out how to take care of all the things that arise, but this, in itself, can contribute to increasing stress in this period of your life. In my opinion, it is important that we choose to include friends as one of the elements in our life, in order to enjoy a happy, healthy, fulfilling retirement.

HEALTH

I have also noticed that, occasionally, people alone will ignore health issues that would be better dealt with early on. When you are alone, you might not get the feedback you need to go look into something that needs attention. I have heard it said that we live life by "choice" or by "default." To me, this means we are called to give conscious attention to a concern, like our health. Waiting until we have symptoms means we've waited until we're in default, and a problem has appeared. This is similar to the advice I gave my dental patients. It is much easier and less expensive to deal with problems if you choose to have frequent checkups and are consciously engaging in good self-care.

So, here's a good plan to adopt:

1.   **Yearly checkups** with your primary care doctor, and see your dentist/hygienist at least every six months.

2.   **Adopt a method of exercise** that involves movement, balance, and strength building. I discovered that my Medicare supplemental insurance policy provides me with a free card that allows me to go to many of the local gyms. In addition, the senior center in my neighborhood has a wonderful array of classes encouraging physical health. There are also a wealth of CDs that you can use to exercise at home. (Several that were highly recommended by users are noted in the Resource Section at the end of the book.)

3.   **Don't ignore symptoms that arise.** If something is bothering you, contact a professional and find out what you need to do.

4.   **Be proactive/add any steps needed** to cover the health problems you might be having.

SO, IS THERE A (PART-TIME) JOB IN MY FUTURE?

On January 17, 2017, *Today* did a show on retirement. The show pointed out that many retirees have chosen to continue working part-time in some capacity and mentioned the beneficial effects that choosing to continue to work can give you:

1.   **It keeps you alive** – Researchers from Oregon State University analyzed data from an ongoing study of people age 50 and up. What they found was that people who continued to work past 65 had an 11 percent lower chance of death from all causes.

2.   It keeps you healthier – Researchers from the University of Miami studied more than 80,000 participants of the National Health Interview Survey, all of whom were at least 65 years old. Thirteen percent were still working. People in the workforce were significantly more likely to report their health was good, very good or excellent than those who were unemployed or retired.

3.   It keeps you mentally sharp – Even people who thought they were doing it for the money came to realize that working improved their mental health. It keeps you connected to people, more current with technology, up to date on the news, and (generally) physically active.

4.   It reduces isolation – Dan Veto, senior advisor to AgeWave, says that isolation, one of the real risks of retirement, is as unhealthy as smoking a pack of cigarettes a day.

5.   It gives you an identity – Work gives you a reason to get up in the morning. We all like to be able to say, "Here's what I do." It gives you a sense of belonging to a unit greater than yourself.

6.   You can delay taking Social Security – In general, every year you don't take your benefits between age 62 and age 70 allows the benefits to grow 8 percent annually.

7.   You may still receive company benefits. For example, your employer's health insurance may be cheaper than Medicare.

As we have discussed, you can achieve these goals with other pursuits. But the point presented in this program is that a large number of people continue to choose part-time work.

A good place to begin this discussion is to guesstimate how much additional income you would like to have coming in. Some people decide to collect these funds with investments, and there is a great deal of information available to assist you in this area. You can also do what Al Hicks did and look for an endeavor where you can utilize your previous job skills.

A number of retirees have reported that their company let them stay on as a consultant. This can be a good option, especially if you like what you have been doing and there is a choice to work as much or as little as you want. This seems especially useful for people who want to continue earning and still have the freedom to take time for other endeavors. It is also a way to ease into retirement, especially for those who aren't quite sure what they are going to do with the rest of their lives. One man told me exactly that: "I would love to retire but I don't have anything else I want to do, so I just keep working."

One family in our neighborhood experienced the need for additional income. One of their sons needed some "seed money" to begin a company, and they loaned it to him from their IRA account. When the company was not a success, they found themselves needing to replace the money for their future retirement. The husband stayed at his job as a consultant for a few more years to ensure that they could continue living at their present level.

Here's a list of some of the interesting part-time jobs I have come across:
- Two friends have taken part-time jobs driving for several companies (Uber and Lyft) that provide taxi service via a cell phone app. When I expressed my concern, I was assured that it has been safe and profitable for them both.
- People who have a house have taken in roommates, with varying results. The most recent extension of this concept is the use of an online company that facilitates rentals for people looking for a vacation option other than motel/ hotel accommodations.

- Retired teachers have taken tutoring jobs.
- One individual is working security at an arena that presents a variety of productions and games (she also gets to see all the entertainment).

I'm sure you could add some examples of your own, of jobs that you have seen friends/family members decide to do.

_____

_____

_____

_____

_____

_____

You may discover that your need for additional income is not so great that it requires a full-time job. A part-time job might be very enjoyable—doing something you might not have considered when you needed full-time work. I have a teacher friend who went to work as a part-time salesclerk at a department store during sales events. She enjoys the discounts that come with the job.

SO . . . IS THERE A PART-TIME JOB . . . FOR ME?

For those of you who might want to entertain the possibility of a part-time job, here's a place to try that on. It's also an opportunity to use the intuitive skills you developed in Chapter 4. Even those of you who aren't sure if you want a job might enjoy this exercise. And . . . you might discover you do want to try something new!

Let this be fun! You can use the criteria we have discussed in previous chapters to experiment with these questions:

*What kind of work would appeal to me at this time?

*What would I love to start to do/do next?

*What are important considerations that would need my attention (time, travel distance, etc.)?

*What new job/career would I attempt if my "logical mind" wasn't busy telling me that I'm too old, I am not strong enough, and money, education, experience, gender, age and time were not factors to be considered and dealt with?

*How can I use the talents/skills I discovered in Chapter 2?

I can just sense that, right about now, some of you are ready to balk. This is definitely a place to let your creative self out to play.

Listing a job that might not turn out to be a definite possibility will give you a chance to look at what you find attractive about working in that arena.

So, let's get busy!

First – On the next page, start a list of jobs you are attracted to.

Next – Spend a few minutes thinking about what attracts you to each job. Make notes about this quality next to the job.

Last – Copy these attractive qualities onto this list and recognize that you have created the kind of job you want to be looking for! Excellent work!

POSSIBLE PART-TIME JOBS FOR ME

_____

_____

_____

_____

_____

_____

_____

Here's an "Extra Credit" question for you:

"If a job is attractive to me, what are the qualities I like about it and what beginning step can I take today that will move me in the direction I want to go?"

While doing the research for this chapter, I couldn't help but notice a pattern emerging. Every one of the "Show Me Da Money" books that pertain to this chapter have one thing in common; they all speak to the essential relationship between money/affluence and gratitude. As an example, here's a quote from Suze Orman, _9 Steps to Financial Freedom: Practical & Spiritual Steps So You Can Stop Worrying._

When you are grateful –
when you can see what you have –
you unlock blessings to flow in your life.
—Suze Orman

HOMEWORK ASSIGNMENT – CHAPTER 5

This is a good place to start a dialogue with yourself about how you view your finances. Surprisingly enough, many people haven't really delved deeply into this subject and, as I mentioned in this chapter, a number of unknowns may come into play.

There are many places to research financial management, so I am not including that information here. But a good plan is to study your feelings and ideas about your financial readiness to face the rest of your life. You will discover whether you feel OK with your present financial plans or if you need to work a little more in this area.

THOUGHTS ABOUT MY FINANCES

_____

_____

_____

_____

_____

_____

_____

_____

CHAPTER 6
PAY IT FORWARD

The meaning of life is to find your gift,
the purpose of life is to give it away.
—David Viscott

IS THERE A SERVICE OPPORTUNITY CALLING ME?

This chapter is about the possibility of using the talents you have amassed through the years to help others and thus "pay it forward." The first time I heard about this philosophy was in the movie of the same name. The principle essentially states that we look at the gifts we are given and, instead of returning the favor to the person who gave us the present in the first place, we pass the giving on to someone else. I found this principle amazing and wonderful; a real and unique opportunity to be a benefactor to someone who wasn't expecting anything. And I have found that if you keep your mind and eyes open, the opportunities will be there.

Ask yourself this question: "Is there a service opportunity calling me?" If the answer is yes, or even maybe, consider the possibility that you are a gift you could be putting to good use, for more than one right reason.

Even in retirement, even when you're only looking
to get off the fast track and "smell the roses,"
you should be pushing past what you merely
enjoy into what has real meaning to you. . .
Without an activity that really matters to you,
you're going to feel empty…
—Barbara Sher

When you make the decision to be of service to someone (or something), you have, once again, the opportunity to put your intuition to work. The first part of this process involves just making the decision to share the unique person you are, and then consciously watching for your chance to appear. I guarantee something will come along that ignites your interest.

What we, as retired seniors, have to contribute to the community is often overlooked. It often seems that members of our society become so involved with their own concerns that seniors become invisible. This is where doing service comes in. Many cultures use their elders and their wisdom and experience to teach the lessons of life. In the United States, it is not uncommon to find many seniors in assisted living homes with only other seniors for company.

During one of her programs, Oprah Winfrey said that we, as human beings, generally want to know the answers to these questions:

Do you see me?
Do you hear me?
Do I matter?

Many seniors find that the response to these questions is, at best, a "maybe, sometimes." As retired seniors, we have amassed wisdom that can be overlooked in the structure of our society.

Let no one ever come to you
without leaving better and happier.
Be the living expression of God's kindness:
kindness in your face,
kindness in your eyes,
kindness in your smile.
—Mother Teresa

My personal philosophy includes sharing the time and talent I have been given and developed over my life. I can truly say that the things I do for others light me up from the inside out. I have discovered many opportunities to help. At the present time, as I've noted, I am drawn to entertaining veterans and other seniors.

Our performing groups, the Sensational Ladies (and a few good men) and Sensational Seniors, put on shows at local senior centers, veterans' homes, fairgrounds and on special occasions, such as Christmas and Veterans Day. You couldn't ask for more appreciative audiences. Our "Salute to the Military" honors each branch of the service and each man and woman present who are veterans with the flag and anthem of their branch of the service, plus cheers and applause.

I have discovered places to apply what life has taught me and found these experiences incredibly enriching and fulfilling. In looking at an adventure that offers me the possibility to be a contributor in some way, I like using some of the items

Mary Morrissey mentions in her book, *Building Your Field of Dreams*. You can use as many of the criteria as you find relevant.

Golden Nuggets Checklist from Mary Morrissey

1. Would this undertaking bring me more aliveness?
2. Is it in alignment with my core values?
3. Would it require me to grow?
4. Do I need help from my Higher Power?
5. Is there good (blessings/gifts) in this for others?

When contemplating beginning something new, ask yourself these questions and listen for the voice of your intuition to reply. Then *choose* from a place of what *you* want to try. Being in service becomes a synergistic adventure when both the giver and receiver are enjoying and benefiting from the experience.

TO WHOM MUCH IS GIVEN

It is not by muscle, speed
or physical dexterity
that great things are achieved,
but by reflection, force of character,
and judgment.
In these qualities old age is usually not poorer, but is even richer.
—Cicero

I remember hearing this Bible verse (Luke 12:48) many years ago and then feeling a sense of responsibility creep over me. I have had a wonderful life in many ways and so, as the verse finishes saying, "much is expected from me." I love the philosophy of these words and decided to paraphrase the quote to say,

"To whom much is given, many opportunities to help are possible."

It feels much more inspiring and, to me, much less like a heavy responsibility.

Mother Teresa is a wonderful example of someone who lived her life fully and in service to others. Not many are called to her complete selflessness, but her example provides wonderful illustrations of how small acts of kindness can be big contributions. She spent twenty years of her life taking care of the sick, poor, and dying. You can also allow yourself to be "called" to be in service to something, someone, or some organization.

Where are you being called . . .?
What has heart and meaning to you?
What would you like to be doing? . . .
What contributions do you want to make?
—Angeles Arrien

The need is all around us. The challenge is to find what calls to you and lights you up. Look for ways you can be helpful and alleviate difficulty for others through your compassion. I never thought that dancing, singing, and acting could be a service, but they truly are.

Face it, we are all living in a "temporary form." I don't see this as depressing but as an encouragement to make the most of and use up my life. For me, this includes being in service. It's as simple as keeping your eyes and ears open to the opportunities that arise. Once you have fallen in love with being in service to others, you no longer need to be encouraged to reach out. I know that is my experience, and I enjoy watching the new opportunities arise.

Mary Ellen Carter, whose story appeared in Chapter 2, saw such an opportunity when she was visiting Malawi with her husband. Over an eight-year period the organization she created, Direct Connections to Africa, has had an amazing effect in the areas of education, health, water provisions and everyday living.

GRATITUDE/FULFILLMENT

Seeing your life through the eyes of gratitude can completely change this time of life. If you were encouraged, as I was, to be a problem solver, you may have developed the habit of looking for what is wrong and what needs to be fixed. This attitude can, occasionally, put a damper on gratitude and happiness. So, as you begin the habit of looking for what you enjoy, appreciate, and love, you will notice you have become thankful for the blessings of your life.

This "attitude of gratitude" is guaranteed to bring you more happiness. You will discover that it opens you to increased generosity and the desire to share the talents you have discovered you possess. Extending this generosity will enrich your life at home, in your community, and in your relationships.

CREATIVITY

This period of your life and the space you have created opens you to explore another aspect of yourself that might have been given a low priority because of the need to make a living and raise a family. Retirement is a wonderful time in which you can unearth past talents you weren't able to make time for and discover exciting new pursuits that will bring you to that place of excitement and joy.

Having joined the Sensational Ladies, I used my free time to work on my acting and singing talents. The people in my group are all over 65, and yet the enthusiasm and excitement we have belies our number of years on the planet.

I would like to call your attention to a book I found to be valuable. It's called *The Artist's Way*, by **Julia Cameron**. It is not a how-to book. Rather, it presents a process that guides you to discover your own creativity and integrate it into who you are and what you want to express. I used the concepts in this book to encourage and guide me into the unknown arenas of acting and singing. One of my favorite exercises is the "artist's date," in which you get to explore this part of you.

Julia Cameron has published a new book, *It's Never Too Late to Begin Again: Discovering Creativity and Meaning at Midlife and Beyond*. It is designed as a twelve-week course and will, I guarantee, create a new awareness of you, in you.

Remember, it is important to include fun, laughter, and play in your life. Being happy contributes to creativity and encourages curiosity and openness to exploring "what's next."

YOUR LEGACY

Sharing your message with any size audience will always be a meaningful act
and a true path to purpose and fulfillment in life.
There is meaning in mentoring others,
and satisfaction in serving.
—Brendon Burchard

What if your legacy was to share the wisdom you've gained (so far!) along your unique life's journey? Imagine what an incredible "pay it forward" that would be!

How you decide to use this period of your life is up to you. I have chosen to squeeze every ounce of everything I love into this time. And it has been, and still is, wonderful! Stephen R. Covey addresses this issue in his book, *The 7 Habits of Highly Effective People.* He discusses this period of life as one in which, "The most important work you will ever do is always ahead of you. It is never behind you. You should always be expanding and deepening your commitment to that work." I found this an exciting concept: the best is yet to come! He calls "retirement" a false concept and declares, "You may retire from a job, but never retire from meaningful projects and contributions."

Stephen Covey further adds, "Regardless of what you have or haven't accomplished, you still have important contributions to make. Avoid the temptation to keep looking in the rearview mirror at what you have done and instead look ahead with optimism." This has been my experience, and I find it is more easily done when in the company of people with the same belief.

DR. JAMES TURRELL'S STORY

I met with Dr. Jim at his office. He is the pastor of the Center for Spiritual Living, Newport-Mesa, as well as a musician, the author of 14 books, a teacher, and a counselor. His personal philosophy reflects a practical approach in a productive and loving way. Dr. Jim says, "To be effective you must be active, creative and engaged."

With his background in counseling, I asked him what he would recommend to a client who was retiring. He said, "Look for a cause that is bigger than yourself and find a way to be in service." Keeping this strategy in mind will allow you to become engaged in a cause that lights you up and uses the skills you have amassed over the years. Many organizations are looking for this kind of assistance. These organizations provide opportunities for you to use the brand of assistance you have to offer. Seniors contribute a wealth of knowledge that is recognized and welcomed in many places. My own personal experience is all about the joy I receive being in service to others.

Dr. Jim's methods involve starting each day with a commitment to live in peace. With this pledge for the day in place, your approach to any event will be dramatically different than if you were just reacting to what came along. It allows you to live your life productively, from a place of choice. For example, if you drive on the freeway in heavy traffic, you can create a different reaction if you have pledged to live in peace that day.

When you commit to a life of peace, your "peripheral vision" expands and activates new opportunities. Instead of narrowly focusing on what is wrong, you see and open up to new opportunities that engage life. Dr. Jim says, "Developing this way of being requires a period of 'research and development'—finding out what personally works for you." This doesn't guarantee everything will go perfectly, but it does help you see your choices from a perspective of what you are wanting to have present in your life. For me, I was able to exist in a more positive way, and it has opened me to many adventures I would never have had if I wasn't seeing life through a "wide-angle lens."

You must look for the opportunities being presented by life, and *take action*. The peripheral vision that led you to this opportunity will help you find the first step . . . and, from there, other steps will appear until you are well on your way.

HOMEWORK ASSIGNMENT – CHAPTER 6

On the lines below, answer and elaborate on these questions/statements:

1. What do I really enthusiastically love to do when I'm with others?

2. How could I use the talents/abilities I discovered in Chapter 1 and Chapter 2 to help others?

3. How can I get into action/what will be a first step?

4. I am grateful/happy knowing that I am able to contribute:

_____

_____

_____

_____

_____

_____

_____

_____

_____

_____

HOW I FEEL ABOUT SHARING MY GIFTS

_____

_____

_____

_____

_____

_____

_____

_____

_____

_____

_____

_____

_____

_____

_____

CHAPTER 7
LIFE HASN'T PASSED ME BY —IT ISN'T DONE WITH ME YET!

I choose to make
the rest of my life,
the best of my life.
—Louise Hay

DREAMING "OUTSIDE THE BOX"

Congratulations! You have completed an in-depth examination of your wonderful life and begun creating your "what's next." After the amount of work you have done so far, I'm sure you see that life hasn't ended; it isn't done with you yet.

Your adventure through this book has allowed you to revisit many aspects of your life up until now. And dream about what still can be out there for you to experience.

You have examined your careers, life roles, etc., and extracted the talents and skills that still remain as a major part of you.

You have dealt with grieving the loss of that part of your life and looked for the possibilities still waiting to be experienced.

The secret of genius
is to carry the spirit
of the child into old age,
which means never
losing your enthusiasm.
—Aldous Huxley

You have "cleaned up" the self-talk you might have been using and discovered the power of your intuition.

You have decided whether you need (or want) to continue working and discovered how to share your talents and gifts with others who could really benefit from all you have to contribute.

REREADING YOUR ANSWERS

So now, let's take this time to reread your answers to the exercises in this book. This is a good way to review the work you have done and make any additions that come to mind. As I mentioned, it has been my experience that new ideas often appear when I revisit a list I have already started. And it's wonderful to take a second look at your process this far and recognize the new realizations you have come to about *you*. All the success you brought into creating your history before retirement is present here and willing to help create this next meaningful time of your life.

Once you have completed this review, you will be ready to take an in-depth look at your Bucket List.

MY BUCKET LIST—DREAMING OUTSIDE THE BOX

To change one's life:
1. Start immediately.
2. Do it flamboyantly.
3. No exceptions.
—William James

Turn back to your Bucket List in Chapter 3, and take a deep look at each item. Add any new possibilities that come to mind. Remember, this isn't set in stone; it's just an opportunity. Let yourself experience the feelings that come up around each potential undertaking. If you find that a certain item has a big impact on you, mark it with a star.

As mentioned before, this is not about logic but about looking at what lights you up, gives you energy. You're now ready to continue moving along the road of your retirement adventure.

TAKING THE FIRST STEP

You don't have to see the whole staircase,
just take the first step.
—Martin Luther King, Jr.

It is now time to begin exploring some of the starred items on your Bucket List. I hope you have found things that light you up and will contribute to this part of your process.

In his book, *The Code of the Extraordinary Mind: 10 Unconventional Laws to Redefine Your Life and Succeed On Your Own Terms,* **Vishen Lakhiani** addresses the importance of taking first/baby steps to manifest your objective. He states that "baby steps show intention. They show that you're standing at attention and ready to receive marching orders. You may not know the optimal path to get to where you're bound to go, but your boots are on and you're going. . . . And something will come of that!"

> *Connecting to intention means*
> *listening to your heart*
> *and conducting yourself*
> *based on what your inner voice*
> *tells you is your purpose here.*
> —Wayne Dyer

On the next page, take the items on the Bucket List that you marked with a star because they resonated with you, and add the possible ways you could "take the first step" into each experience. Use your imagination, even adding things that your logical mind might say are not possible. Although it is not unusual to feel slightly overwhelmed at the prospect of starting anew, of being a beginner again like we talked about earlier, this exercise opens the door to possibilities you might not have even considered. I have also heard it recommended that you find and take the easiest steps first. Once you get going, momentum will keep propelling you along your course.

When I was taking education classes to become a teacher, we were presented with the philosophy that "Success breeds success." I have used that philosophy in my own learning processes and found that, indeed, your confidence increases as you move successfully through each step. I also found that as your determination grows, you become even more daring than you thought you could ever be.

So start working on discovering possible baby steps for your starred Bucket List items. And let your enthusiasm lead you to continue the journey!

FIRST/BABY STEPS

_____

_____

_____

_____

_____

_____

_____

COIN TOSS EXERCISE

When you have finished making note of possible Baby Steps, do this fun exercise.

First: Read over and choose your two favorite items from the list. Give one the designation "heads" and the other the designation "tails." Then toss a coin, and see which one fate has chosen for you.

Next: Sit with fate's decision and examine the feelings that come up. You may be excited and feel that this is, indeed, the perfect first choice . . . or you may find yourself disappointed and decide that the other item is really what you wanted to explore first. Either way, this exercise will be a win-win for you!

As you begin to put the "first step" philosophy into play, read this example of the power of this approach. This is a story about William Murray.

W. H. Murray had survived two prisoner-of-war camps during World War II and made the decision to fulfill a dream of his, that of joining a mountain-climbing party put together by his friend Edmund Hillary. The group planned to climb Mount Everest, and Murray had a deep desire to go.

To join a party like this, people are required to pay their own expenses, an expensive proposition. When Murray found out how much it cost, he realized he didn't have enough money.

The original party didn't make it to the top of the world, so Hillary planned a second climb. He invited Murray on this second trip also. Murray asked again what the cost was going to be. Upon hearing the amount, he realized he couldn't afford this second trip either.

As Hillary planned his third and last trek (he was determined to complete the climb, as he hadn't been able to in the past), he asked Murray, once again, to accompany the party and informed him this would be the last climb he would organize.

Murray was about to ask the same question about the cost, but decided to just inquire about the down payment. When he heard that amount, he realized he could afford to reserve his spot. He went on to do the climb and, this time, the party was able to complete the climb up Mount Everest. He wrote this about what he learned about taking the first step—that of putting a down payment on the trip.

Until one is committed, there is hesitancy, the chance to draw back, always inef-
fectiveness. Concerning all acts of initiative (and creation), there is one elemen-
tary truth the ignorance of which kills countless ideas and splendid plans: that the
moment one definitely commits oneself, then providence moves too.
A whole stream of events issues from the decision, raising in one's favor all manner of
unforeseen incidents, meetings and material assistance,
which no man could have dreamt would have come his way.
I learned a deep respect for one of Goethe's couplets: Whatever you can do or dream
you can, begin it. Boldness has genius, power and magic in it!
—W. H. Murray

MAKING THIS TRANSITION A PRIORITY

I will not waste a moment mourning yesterday's misfortunes, yesterday's defeats,
yesterday's aches of the heart, for why should I throw good after bad?
—Og Mandino

Now is your time to grow your future into what I have discovered is more than could possibly be imagined! What is required now is to make this transition a real priority. Think of the effort you expended to create the first part of your life, and put that wonderful passion to work here. As you take first steps, I guarantee others will present themselves, and you're on your way.

There are a number of places to delve into for inspiration; I have noted a few here and in the Resource Section at the back of the book. If you keep your eyes open and ears alert, you will discover many more. One possibility is to look for any groups/clubs that support an activity that attracts you, or surf the internet to find out where activities in your area might be listed. A list of senior activities is often provided in the newspaper (if you still read one), and look at local senior centers in your area; they often provide an amazing array of chances to develop new skills and interact with other seniors.

You can also check out emeritus programs at local community colleges. I have used the local colleges to study a variety of things, ranging from tap dancing and theater arts to health sciences. These colleges provide excellent teachers, and we make great students. I am sure, with your thinking cap in place, you will discover more possibilities. Everything you try opens doors to new people and new chances to participate in life. This is the time to invest energy in yourself, to spend time making your transition a priority, and to watch for happiness to appear as the adventure continues to reveal itself.

My whole Ms. Senior California experience was a "first step." That led me to the Sensational Ladies, a group of women (and a few good men) who continue to inspire me "to be more than I thought I could be." In 2016, we traveled as far as New Orleans to perform at the Mardi Gras and to Las Vegas and Laughlin, Nevada, to do shows. We're also getting ready to start rehearsals on a musical, "Cinemagic," based on movie songs through the years.

I choose to risk . . .
to live so that which came to me
as seed goes to the next as a blossom,
and that which came to me as a blossom,
goes on as fruit.
—Dawna Markova

THOUGHT OF THE DAY

Don't waste this precious day creating regrets. Invest your time creating value.

Don't work against your own interests by using your energy to feel sorry for yourself. You can use that same energy, and more, to get beyond whatever may be troubling you.

The choices you make are what determine the quality of the life you live. Every time you have a choice to make, you have the opportunity to make life richer and more fulfilling.

You are immersed in abundance and possibility. Have the presence of mind to see it, and have the courage to make the most of it all.

There's no limit to the number of ways you can make a difference. Remind yourself of that, and remind yourself of all that truly matters to you.

The opportunity is yours, and it is called "Life."

Now live it well!

—Ralph S. Marston, Jr.

The Daily Motivator, http://greatday.com/

RESOURCE SECTION

Give yourself permission to live your life to the fullest, whatever that looks and feels like to you.

The listings below are provided to present possible adventures to enhance the new you in your new life.

ARE YOU LOOKING TO LAUNCH YOUR RETIREMENT BY LEARNING AT HOME?

The Great Courses: Offers the best of the best college-level courses on CD, DVD, and digital formats. Over 500 expertly produced courses by professors chosen for their ability to teach. Investigate this site to see the wonderful selection of subjects . . . and, no homework. www.thegreatcourses.com/

DO YOU WANT TO MAKE NEW FRIENDS?

Senior Centers: Look into the senior center in your area. These centers typically provide a wonderful array of classes, an opportunity to meet others, and lunch at a reasonable price.

THINKING ABOUT WRITING A BOOK?

Everyone has a story to tell and ideas to share. The **CSL Writer's Workshop** makes it possible for you to stop thinking and start writing. This program provides 24-hour online access to all class videos. You learn to choose your subject, create your title, write a paragraph that identifies the problem your book will solve, and generate your chapter titles. Then, using the timed writing exercises, you can write your rough draft during the class sessions. Learn how professional writers create an emotional connection with the reader. You also learn to edit what you've written and construct a marketing plan to sell your book. For more information go to www.CSLWritersWorkshop.com

LOOKING FOR CLASSES DESIGNED FOR SENIORS?

Community College Emeritus Classes: Check out your local community colleges and universities for courses offered for older people with the intention to "promote lifelong learning by providing classes that are academically rigorous, mentally stimulating, socially engaging and designed to improve/maintain health."

LOOKING TO GET INTO SHAPE?

Silver Sneakers Card: May be provided by your Medicare Supplemental Insurance plan; mine was. It allows me to attend many of the top gyms for free. Call your supplemental insurance company to see if it provides this service.

LOOKING TO GET IN SHAPE AT HOME?

A number of CDs can be ordered from Amazon.com. Here are several that were rated high by users:

Stronger Seniors® Stretch and Strength DVDs: Two-disc Chair Exercise Program – Stretching, Aerobics, Strength Training, and Balance. Improve flexibility, muscle and bone strength, circulation, heart health, and stability. Developed by Anne Pringle Burnell.

Discover Tai Chi for Balance and Mobility (Scott Cole Wellness Series)

Absolute Beginners—Cardio and Strength Training Workout for Seniors

WANT TO TAKE A HIKE?

Sierra Club Seniors: This program offers many different outings, from docent-led museum and gallery tours to challenging Sierra hikes. The program welcomes all seniors who are interested in conservation and wish to participate in the activities listed on the group's Facebook Page.

DO YOU WANT TO FIND PEOPLE WHO LIKE TO DO THE SAME THINGS YOU DO?

Seniors Meetups: Designed to help you meet other seniors in your local area! These clubs cover a wide variety of activities. This is one of the sites I found online. You can find others that target specific activities.

Seniors Meetups - https://www.meetup.com/topics/seniors/

LOOKING TO LET YOUR ARTIST OUT INTO ACTION?

Julia Cameron has classes available both online and at certain sites. Her process is very helpful for getting started. Visit http://juliacameronlive.com/the-artists-way/ to see what's coming up in your area. This is a wonderful way to develop a new hobby.

WANT TO FIND A MULTITUDE OF ACTIVITIES IN YOUR AREA?

City Parks and Recreation Departments: Many cities offer a variety of classes through the Parks and Recreation Department. I checked with my city and discovered it is possible to brush up on computer programs, take cooking classes, learn photography and other art forms, pick up any of a number of dance techniques and exercise modalities, train a dog, etc. The classes are provided for a nominal fee.

WANT TO TAKE A TRIP?

A number of companies provide travel programs at good rates for seniors. Most recently, I have used:

Gate 1 Travel—This company offers a wide selection of escorted tours and independent air and hotel packages, so you have a choice of destination and travel style. Check out what it has to offer at: Tourvacationstogo.com/gate_1_travel.cfm

Road Scholar.org—(used to be Elderhostel) This company provides information about hundreds of "learning adventures" by location or interest. They offer "Inspiring instructors, spirited conversations, new friends, new experiences — being a Road Scholar encompasses the best of the university experience."

Viator Tours—I used it to book destination tours and found it reasonable and helpful. I found it helpful to have my tours arranged before I left on vacation to better plan the time I have in a certain location. www.Viator.com.

LOOKING FOR A PET?

If you feel ready for a "fur friend," many rescue organizations place animals looking for a forever family. Among them: **Pet Expos**, your local **Animal Shelter,** and pet stores that offer pets for adoption. Some organizations place specific breeds.

LOOKING TO HELP SOMEONE WHO NEEDS WHAT YOU HAVE TO OFFER?

A multitude of nonprofit organizations are looking for volunteers. Try out a few and see which one sparks your fancy. Review the talents you have identified and find a place that can use you.

RECOMMENDED READING LIST

The selections in this list are here to be of greater service to you in any area where you may want additional support and guidance. Authors whose names are bolded here are also quoted in this book.

> *Let go of what no longer serves you*
> *by embracing what does.*
> —Dennis Merritt Jones

Dennis Merritt Jones. *The Art of Being: 101 Ways to Practice Purpose in Your Life.* Simi Valley, CA: New Reality Press, 2004.

Dennis Merritt Jones. *The Art of Uncertainty: How to Live in the Mystery of Life and Love It.* New York: Tarcher/Perigee, 2011.

> *People arrive to help us in our darkest hours . .*
> *someone we might never [otherwise] have met,*
> *ends up giving us pivotal assistance . . .*
> —Marianne Williamson

Marianne Williamson. *Tears to Triumph: The Spiritual Journey from Suffering to Enlightenment.* New York: HarperCollins, 2016.

Marianne Williamson. *The Gift of Change: Spiritual Guidance for Living Your Best Life.* New York: HarperCollins, 2004.

*Even in retirement, even when you're only looking to
get off the fast track and "smell the roses,"
you should be pushing past what you merely enjoy into what has real meaning to you.
Without an activity that really matters to you, you're going to feel empty . . .*
—Barbara Sher

Barbara Sher. *I Could Do Anything If Only I Knew What It Was: How to Discover What You Really Want and How to Get It.* New York: Dell, 1994.

*Connecting to intention means listening to your heart and conducting yourself based
on what your inner voice tells you is your purpose here.*
—Wayne Dyer

Dr. Wayne Dyer. *The Power of Intention: Learning to Co-create Your World Your Way.* Carlsbad, CA: Hay House, 2004.

*I choose to make the rest of my life
the best of my life.*
—Louise Hay

Louise Hay. *You Can Heal Your Life.* Carlsbad, CA: Hay House, 1987, 1999.

*Sometimes you have to destroy a part of your life
to let the next thing enter.*
—Vishen Lakhiani

Vishen Lakhiani. *The Code of the Extraordinary Mind: 10 Unconventional Laws to Redefine Your Life & Succeed on Your Own Terms.* New York: Rodale Books, 2016.

> *Where are you being called . . . ? What has heart*
> *and meaning for you? What would you like to be doing? . . .*
> *What contributions do you want to make?*
> —Angeles Arrien

Angeles Arrien. *The Second Half of Life: Opening the Eight Gates of Wisdom.* Boulder, CO: Sounds True, 2007.

> *Living a life of love and service. . . isn't a quick fix. But it's possible.*
> *It begins with the desire to center our lives on correct principles,*
> *to break out of . . . the comfort zones of unworthy habits.*
> —Stephen R. Covey

Stephen R. Covey. *The 7 Habits of Highly Effective People: Powerful Lessons in Personal Change.* New York: Simon & Schuster, 1989, 2013.

> *As a friend of mine worried recently, "All I do is work.*
> *When I stop working, will I do . . . nothing?'"*
> *The answer is no.*
> —Julia Cameron

Julia Cameron. *It's Never Too Late to Begin Again: Discovering Creativity and Meaning at Midlife and Beyond.* New York: Random House, 2016.

Julia Cameron. *The Artist's Way: A Spiritual Path to Higher Creativity.* New York: Tarcher/Putnam, 1992, 2002.

Sometimes we have built the walls ourselves, but often it's the nature of things that walls that once served and sheltered us at certain periods of our life only imprison us when we have remained within their confines for too long.
—David Whyte

David Whyte. *Crossing the Unknown Sea: Work as a Pilgrimage of Identity.* New York: Penguin, 2002.

Rather than being driven by what you've been missing, it's more powerful to intentionally identify all the elements you truly desire, which will support your well-being.
—John E. Nelson, in *65 Things to Do When You Retire*

Mark Evan Chimsky, Ed. *65 Things to Do When You Retire.* South Portland, ME: Sellers, 2012

*I choose to risk . . . to live so that which came to me
as seed goes to the next as a blossom, and that
which came to me as a blossom, goes on as fruit.*
—Dawna Markova

Dawna Markova. *I Will Not Die an Unlived Life: Reclaiming Purpose and Passion.* San Francisco: Red Wheel/Weiser, 2000.

Gregg Braden. *Resilience from the Heart: The Power to Thrive in Life's Extremes.* Carlsbad, CA: Hay House, 2015.

Wealth consciousness, by definition, is a state of mind. Gratitude and generosity are natural attributes of an affluent consciousness.
—Deepak Chopra

Deepak Chopra. *Creating Affluence: The A-to-Z Steps to a Richer Life.* San Rafael, CA: Amber-Allen, 1998.

I will not waste a moment mourning yesterday's misfortunes, yesterday's defeats, yesterday's aches of the heart, for why should I throw good after bad?
—Og Mandino

Dave Blanchard. *Today I Begin a New Life: Intentional Creation: Og Mandino for the 21st Century.* OgPress, 2012.

Sharing your message with any size audience will always be a meaningful act and a true path to purpose and fulfillment in life.
There is meaning in mentoring others, and satisfaction in serving.
—Brendon Burchard

Brendon Burchard. *The Millionaire Messenger: Make a Difference and a Fortune Sharing Your Advice.* New York: Simon & Schuster, 2011.

Mary Morrissey. *No Less Than Greatness: Finding Perfect Love in Imperfect Relationships.* New York: Bantam Books, 2001.

Mary Morrissey. *Building Your Field of Dreams.* New York: Bantam Books, 2013.

ADDITIONAL READING SELECTIONS

Mark Victor Hansen & Art Linkletter. *How to Make the Rest of Your Life the Best of Your Life.* Nashville, TN: Thomas Nelson, 2006.

Marlo Thomas. *It Ain't Over: Reinventing Your Life and Realizing Your Dreams Anytime, at Any Age.* New York: Simon and Schuster, 2014.

Mary & Ronald Hulnick. *Remembering the Light Within: A Course in Soul-Centered Living.* Carlsbad, CA: Hay House, 2017.

Sandra Haldeman Martz, ed. *Grow Old Along with Me—The Best Is Yet to Be.* Watsonville, CA: Papier-Mache Press, 1996.

Edwene Gaines. *The Four Spiritual Laws of Prosperity: A Simple Guide to Unlimited Abundance.* New York: Burke/Triolo, 2005.

Suze Orman. *9 Steps to Financial Freedom: Practical & Spiritual Steps So You Can Stop Worrying.* New York: 3 Rivers Press, 1997, 2012.

ABOUT THE AUTHOR

Ginni Gordon is a pro at retiring! She gives herself permission to live life to the fullest. Before retiring she:

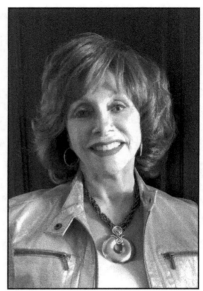

- Married her high school sweetheart, had four children, and attended college. She has five grandchildren; one is in heaven.
- Spent 25 years as a Dental Hygienist (in practice with her dentist/brothers, Larry and Jim Rizzo, in Huntington Beach).
- Taught in the Dental Schools at both the University of Southern California and the University of California, Los Angeles.
- Taught Health Science and Human Service Classes at both Cerritos College and Saddleback College.
- Ran education groups for 20 years for parents of children with drug, alcohol and eating disorder problems.

After retirement (in 2002), her life has been equally exciting! She:

- Learned to act and sing and she has taken her dancing skills into several plays and musicals. She now performs with a group called "Sensational Seniors" that, in the year 2016, performed in New Orleans for Mardi Gras, Las Vegas and Laughlin, Nevada. This group also entertains local seniors, veterans and at county fairs.

- Is a Licensed Practitioner for the Center for Spiritual Living;
- Teaches "Conscious Aging" Workshops;
- Is actively involved in a number of charities; her two favorites are:
  - o Gold Rush Cure Foundation (Her daughter and son-in-law, who lost their son to leukemia, started this organization that mentors and gives gifts to children diagnosed with cancer and works for research cures.)
  - o Direct Connections to Africa (Mary Ellen Carter developed this organization that educates children, provides water wells, health education, etc. for an area in Malawi, Africa. Her story is a featured interview in Chapter 2 of this book.)

And her favorite animal is Lola, a loving and lovable Maltipoo.

CPSIA information can be obtained
at www.ICGtesting.com
Printed in the USA
LVHW01s1210201217
560366LV00018B/826/P

9 780692 901526